I0059940

Atopic Dermatitis.

Understanding Atopic Dermatitis as a disease and
learning how to cope with it through preventative
and curative methods.

by

Robert Rymore

ALL RIGHTS RESERVED. This book contains material protected under International and Federal Copyright Laws and Treaties.

Any unauthorized reprint or use of this material is strictly prohib-
ited. No part of this book may be reproduced or transmitted in any
form or by any means, electronic, mechanical or otherwise, including photocopying or recording, or by any information storage
and retrieval system without express written permission from the
author.

Copyrighted © 2014

Published by: IMB Publishing

Table of Contents

Table of Contents

Table of Contents

Preface

Our skin is the reflection of our image through which we achieve a unique identity in society. Skin is so smooth in its function that we hardly notice the metabolic processes that are going on 24/7.

We notice it most when it develops annoying symptoms. It is said that a ton of pain is more tolerable than a simple itch of the skin. Today, increasing pollutants in the environment and chemicals we encounter in day-to-day life, changing lifestyles and junk food have had a definite impact on skin health. These changes have increased the incidences of various types of skin diseases; among the most common is dermatitis, in the forms of allergic dermatitis, contact dermatitis or urticaria, in addition to others.

Hypersensitivity of the immune system affects the skin and leads to one of the most embarrassing and annoying diseases, contact dermatitis. In this book we have incorporated each and every minute detail about Atopic Dermatitis and answer all your questions, including those that have gone unanswered until now.

Acknowledgements

My special thanks to my wife and my family, who always motivated me to do something different, and all the love and positivity they give me. Without their support it wouldn't be possible to give 100% to this book.

Thank you all.

Chapter 1: An introduction to Atopic Dermatitis

The term "atopic" is derived from Greek literature, and means "strange." The term "dermatitis" means inflammation of the skin. The term "eczema" is used for all types of inflammation of the skin and therefore Atopic Dermatitis is generally referred to as "eczema." Atopic Dermatitis is long lasting and the most severe form of eczema and is a commonly found skin disorder that requires frequent treatment. To better understand the disease, we need to know a few details about skin structure and the function of the skin. Though it will look bit technical, it is important in order to get a comprehensive idea of the disease.

1. Overview of the Anatomy and Physiology of Skin

Skin covers an area of about 20 square feet on the body. It is the largest and the most superficial organ of the body and is the only organ in the human body that covers the whole body. The deeper organs of the body are shielded due to the protective barrier of the skin. Besides protection, the body's temperature is regulated by skin, which allows it to register sensations like heat and cold.

The healthy look of the skin is determined by the coordinated function of all of its structures. If any structure or function of the skin is modified, then the appearance of the skin is altered. For long lasting good appearance and for healthy functioning of the skin, it must be protected from harmful agents. The skin must be given proper nutrition to delay the process of ageing. To provide good skin protection and nutrition, an individual must understand its structure, function and components.

THE LAYERS OF HUMAN SKIN

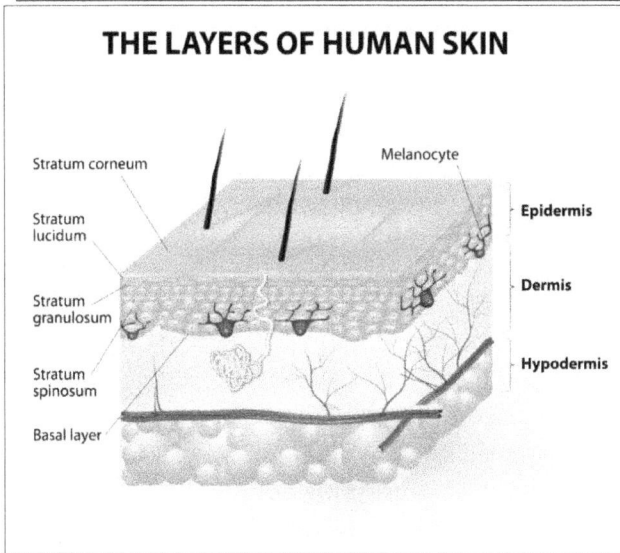

The three components of the skin include:

1) The outermost layer of the skin, which is the epidermis. It is a protective and visible layer of the skin, which is waterproof. Skin tone is determined on the basis of the melanin pigments present in the epidermis. Connective tissue, hair follicles, sweat glands and sebum glands are all found in the epidermis.

2) The dermis is located beneath the epidermis. The dermis is the middle layer of the skin. It provides structure and support to the skin. Connective tissue, hair follicles, sweat glands and sebum glands are also found in the dermis.

3) Beneath the dermis is the hypodermis. It is not a visible layer of the skin. It is deeper, subcutaneous (just below the skin) tissue that consists of fat and connective tissue.

Epidermis

The outermost layer of the skin is known as the epidermis. It is about 0.1 mm in thickness and forms a coating all over the body. It acts as a protective layer for the body and forms a barrier between environmental surroundings and deeper structures. It is categorized into five horizontal layers. In certain places the epidermis may be thick or thin. In thick areas, 100 cell layers are found and in thin areas, 50 cell layers are found. The cells of the epidermis are shed every 28 days and new cells replace the old cells.

The first layer of the epidermis is the stratum basale. It is the deepest structure of the superficial layer of the skin, and is a single layer. It is found exactly above the dermis layer. The cells in the stratum basale are cube shaped. As the epidermal cells are renewed every 28 days, the new cells, which continuously replace the old cells, are known as keratinocytes. These keratinocytes are formed in the stratum basale layer by cell division. This whole process of shedding old cells and forming new cells is known as skin cell renewal. This regenerative process decreases with age.

With age, the dead cells accumulate in the epidermis. Hence, to delay the ageing process the skin cell renewal process should continue for a long time. The stratum basale also consists of melanocytes. Melanocytes produce melanin, which determines the complexion of the skin. With increased melanin, the complexion of the skin is darker. With less melanin, the complexion is fairer. Melanin also provides protection against harmful UVA and UVB rays of the sun. They are potoprotective. Fair-skinned people are more allergic to sunrays due to less melanin found in their skin, whereas dark-skinned people can tolerate sun more and do not suffer from rashes, itching, pigmentation and papules caused by harmful sunrays. Melanin produced by melanocytes is transferred to keratinocytes. Keratinocytes move upwards and the complexion of the skin is maintained evenly.

The second layer of the epidermis is the stratum spinosum. It is also known as the prickle-cell layer. The keratinocytes form the stratum spinosum layer. The keratinocytes are polygonal in shape and usually 10 layers are found. Keratinocytes start converting flat in this layer.

The third layer of the epidermis is known as the stratum granulosum. It is also known as the granular layer. It contains a protein known as keratin. Three to five layers of flat keratin are typically found here. Keratin protein gives the skin its protective properties. Keratin is tough and fibrous in nature. Stratum granulosum has no blood supply as it is not distantly located, nor does it receive blood supply through diffusion. Hence the cells die and are shed away.

The fourth layer of the epidermis is known as the stratum lucidum. It is also known as the clear layer where flat cells are found. Stratum lucidum is found in three to five layers on fingertips, palms, and the soles of the feet.

The fifth layer of the epidermis is known as stratum corneum. It is also known as the horny layer. It is the outermost layer of the epidermis. Stratum corneum provides protection against various harmful agents. It consists of 25-30 layers of dead keratinocytes. Flattened keratinocytes are found here. Dead keratinocytes are shed off and are replaced by new cells. The ceramides, fatty acids, and lipids form the epidermal lipids, which are found in between the keratinocytes. They provide the connecting link between the skin cells. The keratinocytes and the epidermal lipids combine to form a moisture barrier. This is a waterproof layer. It reduces moisture loss from the transepidermal layer of the skin. Moisture is necessary to provide protection against various pathogens, irritants, allergens, heat and cold. The skin becomes extremely dry if the natural moisture barrier is hampered. Severe dryness leads to itching, burning, stinging, redness and cracks on the skin. The skin becomes prematurely old due to lack of moisture and the ageing process occurs faster and wrinkles appear on the skin early. Toxins accumulate and the skin looks unhealthy.

A mild acidic pH level is found in the outermost layer of the epidermis. The pH level ranges from 4.5 to 6.5. This mildly acidic pH is known as the acid mantle. This acid pH is due to sebum secreted from sebaceous glands and sweat secreted from the sweat glands. The acidic environment provides protection against the various pathogens like bacteria, viruses and fungi. They are not able to grow freely in an acidic environment. The acidic mantle of the moisture barrier also maintains the hardness of the keratin. The keratin proteins are firmly bound together due to this hardness.

The alkaline nature of the skin makes the keratin proteins soft and loose. Soft, loose keratin cannot provide toughness for the skin and hence it remains unprotected against daily wear and tear. The alkaline medium is created by the use of low quality soaps, cosmetics and external applications, which disrupt the normal acidic pH of the skin. Due to alkaline pH, the skin becomes rough, dehydrated and irritated. White flakes and scales are seen on the skin. Cracks may be noticed in severe alkaline conditions. The most harmful effect of alkaline pH is easy growth of microorganisms. Boils, furuncles, acne, pimples, etc. occur on the skin as a result of the growth of microorganisms.

Pores, hairs, sebaceous glands, and sweat glands are the components that are found both in the dermis and epidermis layer.

The epidermis layer folds into the dermis layer and leads to pore formation. The pore is lined by the keratinocytes, which grow and shed off in the skin cell renewal process. The process is similar to the topmost layer of the epidermis. The keratinocytes shed from the surroundings of the pore mix with the sebum secreted from the sebaceous glands. This mixture blocks and clogs the pores. When these clogged pores become infected with microorganisms, it gives rise to acne, pimples and boils. The pores become larger and clearly visible when the cells surrounding the pores become irritated and agitated. If oil clogs the pores, they also become enlarged.

The pores open on the surface of the skin. The pores give rise to hairs that are formed of keratin proteins. A bulb-like follicle is found at the base of each hair. The follicle divides and forms new cells. Hairs are dead but the follicle has a blood supply and hence gets nourishment in the form of oxygen and minerals. Hairs on the skin serve as a protective barrier. Minor physical injuries are tolerated by the skin due to the presence of these hairs. The hairs help to retain heat in the body in cold weather. The skin is also protected against the harmful effects of the sun as the hairs block sunrays.

Sebaceous glands are found closely related to the hair follicles. They secrete sebum and oil. The skin and the hair follicles remain moistened and lubricated due to sebum and oil secreted by the glands. Sebum also increases the lipid and the fatty acid level found in the moisture barrier of the skin. The hormone testosterone and other androgens regulate the oil secreted by the sebum glands.

Sweat glands are tabular structures. The cells are longer in size, coiled and hollow. Sweat is produced in the coiled section of the cells. The longer portion of the cell acts as a duct, connecting the gland and the pore that opens on the surface of the skin. Perspiration helps in regulating body temperature.

The body is not heated above the core temperature in normal circumstances, due to the release of sweat from the body. Cooling is maintained and the body is not dehydrated. Sweat also releases harmful toxins from the body. If these toxins are not eliminated via sweat then they accumulate in the body, which leads to various diseases. Sweat also helps in maintaining the acidic pH of the skin.

Dermis

The second layer of the skin is the dermis, which is located in between the deeper hypodermis and the superficial epidermis. The average thickness of the dermis is about 2 mm, but it may vary from person to person. The main function of the dermis is to provide structure to the skin. It is composed of protein, blood vessels that supply the skin, lymph vessels draining the skin, mast cells, fibroblasts, glycosaminoglycan molecules, and more. All

13

these components work together and form a mesh-like network. Protein is found in the form of collagen and elastin. Glycosaminoglycan molecules form the ground substance of the skin, which is a gel-like material that surrounds proteins, blood vessels, lymph vessels, mast cells and other cells of the dermis layer. The natural moisture level of the skin is determined by the ground substance. It also provides a supportive base to various structures of the dermis layer.

The collagen protein is abundantly found in the dermis layer. It is formed of the fibers that appear mesh-like and interlocked with each other. The skin has the necessary strength and flexibility due to the presence of collagen fibres in the dermis layer. The collagen fibres retain the necessary moisture in the skin with the help of glycosaminoglycan molecules (water binding molecules) found in the ground substance. Hence the skin does not become dehydrated and dry. The elastin protein is also abundantly found in the dermis layer. It has a coil-like structure. The elasticity of the skin is attributed to the presence of elastin proteins.

The skin performs various stretching and contracting work daily. After stretching, the skin returns to its normal shape and size due to the presence of elastin protein. If elastin and collagen were not present in the skin, it would not have enough strength to resist routine jerks, shocks and damage. The skin becomes rigid in the absence of these proteins and normal movement is not possible.

Fibroblast cells produce collagen and elastin proteins. Fibroblasts are located on the upper side of the dermis layer just below the epidermis. They form the upper border of the dermis layer.

The blood vessels supplying the skin, lymph vessels that drain the skin, nerves, and mast cells surround and pass between collagen and elastin fibres. Mast cells are also known as allergic cells. They determine the inflammatory response of the skin. The skin reacts to external and internal stimuli due to these specialized cells. The skin encounters various allergens, microorganisms, physical injuries and other irritants daily. Inflammation is triggered by mast cells as a response against these harmful agents and hence the skin and the body remain protected against them.

The blood vessels found in the dermis consist of superficial arteries, veins and capillaries. Blood vessels are not found in the epidermis layer, which is a dead layer, as it has no blood vessels. It lacks oxygen supply and nutrition. Blood vessels supplying the dermis provide very little nutrition to the bottom layers of the epidermis. The blood carries oxygen and nutrition to the cells of the dermis. Without blood supply, the cells and tissues die. The fresh, oxygenated blood is carried through arteries. The deoxygenated blood and the waste products produced by the cells are carried away by veins in the dermis layer. The minute capillaries reach the topmost layer of the dermis, where they diffuse blood supply to the bottom layers of the epidermis.

The blood vessels found in the dermis layer help in maintaining the thermal stability of the body. In the case of extreme cold, the blood vessels constrict and retain the body's heat. In case of extreme heat, the blood vessels dilate and release heat. Thus the body's temperature is maintained.

Dermal papillae are projected structures that are found in between the dermis and epidermis. They are located at the junction of both structures of the skin. They form a wave-like border and provide a medium for the exchange of blood, oxygen and nutrients between the two layers. The surface area for exchange is increased with the help of dermal papillae. These dermal papillae reduce in surface area and become flat as a person's age increases. The exchange of blood and oxygen to the epidermis is also greatly reduced as age increases. Hence the skin looks dehydrated, lusterless, pale and malnourished in old age.

Hypodermis

The hypodermis is a subcutaneous layer just below the skin. It is the deepest structure of the skin, which contains fatty tissues. Fatty tissues determine the thermal balance of the body. The core temperature of the body differs from the outside temperature. For the normal functioning of the body's organs, and to maintain adequate blood flow to all its organs, the body's core temperature must remain at 98.4 degrees Fahrenheit. If the core temperature falls below this normal value, this is known as hypothermia, and if it increases it is termed hyperthermia, or fever.

In hypothermia, the functioning of the organs becomes lethargic and the blood supply is reduced. In hyperthermia, the functioning of the organs increases and flushing of blood may be seen. Toxin production increases in hyperthermia. Hence, the normal core temperature of the body must be maintained, in which the fat cells located in the hypodermis play a very important role. Fat cells in the hypodermis protect the body against bitter winters. It serves as an insulating layer against cold winds, cold water and cold surroundings. It also provides protection against frostbite. (Frostbite occurs when a person steps in snow or freezing cold water for an extended period of time. The blood supply to the lower limbs stops due to the constriction of blood vessels, which leads to necrosis and death of the tissues and the cells.) Very thin people do not possess enough fat cells in the hypodermis layer and hence they feel colder in comparison to larger people.

Fat cells present in the hypodermis are the storehouse of energy. The fat consumed in food is stored in the fat cells of the hypodermis. Energy is released from fat cells when the carbohydrates in the body have been exhausted. The hypodermis serves as a supportive layer between the skin and muscles. It absorbs normal shocks and prevents injury to muscles, deep blood vessels, bones and organs. The hypodermis also provides shape for the body.

The structure of the human body seems attractive and appealing due to the presence of the hypodermis layer. The buttocks, palms of the hands, and soles of the feet have the thickest hypodermis layer. These sites suffer maximum wear and tear while walking, sitting, working and performing other routine work. These sites are therefore well padded by the hypodermis layer so that injury does not occur. The hypodermis also determines the thickness of the skin. People who are very slim have fewer fat cells in the hypodermis and their skin looks thin. People with wasting disorders (disorders which are caused by lack of nutrition) also suffer from loose, elastic and thin skin due to atrophy of the hypodermis layer.

The atrophy of the skin and the hypodermis layer is also seen in old age, which leads to loose, thin, dehydrated, wrinkled and lusterless skin. To delay the ageing process and to prevent the atrophy of the fat cells in the hypodermis layer, a balanced amount of fat in the form of oil, butter, milk and milk products, cheese, clarified butter, etc. must be consumed.

When all the layers of the skin work in a coordinated manner, no skin disease is found. But when any structure of the skin is altered and the normal functioning is hampered, skin diseases can arise.

It is frequently seen that people suffering from Atopic Dermatitis are more concerned about their children getting it, too, and many other questions arise in their mind related to their complaint. In this book we have tried to answer all those questions; those you might have hesitated to ask your skin specialist, or those nobody paid attention to even after asking, such as:

2. Is Atopic Dermatitis a Hereditary Disease and What Does it Commonly Look Like?

The disease may be inherited and is commonly found in first relatives of an affected individual. However, individuals may suffer from the disease without any family history. Individuals suffering from Atopic Dermatitis usually have a personal or family history of asthma or allergic conditions like hay fever, allergic rhinitis and chronic dermatitis.

It has a very typical appearance on the skin where the rashes of the disease may cover the whole body or some parts of the body. The skin is itchy, inflamed, red, swollen, dry, cracked, oozing, crusty, and scaly with blister and vesicle formation. The most common complaints are of dry, red and extremely itchy skin.

3. How Common is Atopic Dermatitis?

Atopic Dermatitis is a commonly found disease and its prevalence is increasing day by day. It can develop at any age, but it commonly affects more infants and children than adults. As age progresses, the onset and severity of the disease is decreased. It is estimated by researchers and doctors that 65% of patients with Atopic Dermatitis have full-fledged symptoms in the first year and 90% of patients have symptoms before the age of five years.

Onset or severity of the disease after 30 years of age is not commonly found. Elderly people are affected with it due to excessive use of harsh chemical agents and exposure to constant, wet surroundings. Individuals dwelling in industrial, polluted and urban areas are prone to having Atopic Dermatitis. A climate of low humidity and dry atmosphere favors the development of Atopic Dermatitis.

Statics on the Prevalence of Atopic Dermatitis:

According to the data available, 15 million people in the United States (approximately 9% -30% of the total population) suffer from Atopic Dermatitis. It affects both males and females in equal proportions. It is estimated that 10% of all infants and young children in the world suffer from Atopic Dermatitis. Among those affected children, approximately 60% of them continue to have few episodes of Atopic Dermatitis until they reach adulthood.

4. Which Famous Personalities have Suffered from Eczema?

Many famous personalities have suffered from eczema in their childhood and have overcome the disease with a little precaution and care.

Leanne Rimes suffered from eczema and psoriasis in her childhood. She admitted in an interview that she was made fun of in school and her peers use to call her "scaly girl." She used to wear full-length clothes so that she could hide her scaling skin. She has admitted that she used to avoid the activities that required her to wear short clothes. She used to avoid swimming in her childhood so that harsh water could not irritate her skin. She could not be involved in her favorite activities as she was restricted due to her lesions, and had to take many precautions. Moreover, she has also said that her mother and father used to apply layers of steroid cream on her whole body day and night.

Britney Spears suffered from foot eczema. Her eczema was aggravated due to stress, overload and the pressure of work.

Nicole Kidman suffered from eczema on her hands, which made them dry, red, scaly, flaky and wrinkled. These skin lesions were clearly visible in her many photographs. She has attended many events and premiers of her movies with eczema on her hands.

Kate Middleton suffered from "atopy" disorders in her childhood and presently is also sensitive to many allergens, especially horse skin. Contact with horse skin triggers sneezing, a runny nose, eczema and asthma in her. Kate was made fun of and was bullied in her school days due to scaly skin and eczema. She was very self-conscious about her skin condition.

Jade Jagger suffered from skin eczema, for which she preferred alternative treatment therapy like homoeopathy.

Brad Pitt also suffered from "contact eczema" due to overuse of cosmetic products. His eczema was aggravated due to the use of harsh, synthetic soaps and cosmetics so he started using only homemade soaps and cosmetics.

Adele suffered from "contact eczema" due to contact with her baby's feeding bottles.

Chapter 2: What Is The Difference Between Atopic Dermatitis and Eczema?

Eczema is a generalized term used for various types of dermatitis (inflammation of skin). Atopic Dermatitis is usually referred to as eczema. Atopic Dermatitis is the chronic and most severe form of eczema.

The other conditions that are referred as eczema include the following:

1) Allergic eczema

2) Contact eczema

3) Seborrhoea eczema

4) Nummular eczema

5) Lichen planus chronicus

6) Stasis dermatitis

7) Dyshidrotic eczema

8) Xerotic eczema

The above conditions are very similar to Atopic Dermatitis and are not easily differentiated. "Atopy" is a term used for a trio of conditions including Atopic Dermatitis, hay fever, and asthma. They may occur together in an individual form or sometimes one condition may flare up and others remain dormant.

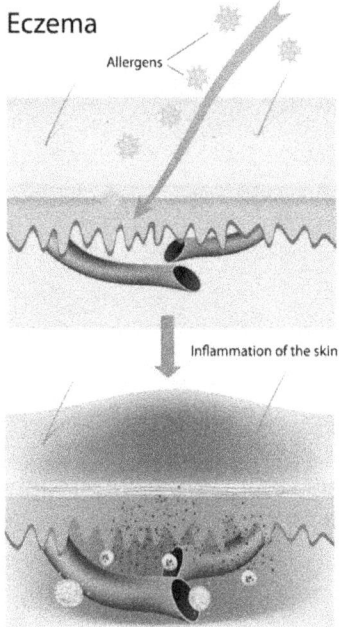

Eczema

Allergens

Inflammation of the skin

Types of eczema:

Contact eczema

This is a localized reaction that occurs when the skin comes into contact with irritating agents such as chemicals, acids, harsh soaps, cleansing agents, etc. Signs and symptoms like redness, itching, and burning occur.

Allergic contact eczema

This is a reaction that occurs when the skin comes into contact with poison ivy, preservatives present in cream, Neosporin or bacitracin lotion, etc. Upon contact with these substances, a foreign body reaction is released by the immune system. Signs and symptoms like redness, itching and oozing occur.

Seborrheic eczema

This is a mild skin inflammation of unknown cause. It is also known as seborrheic dermatitis, seborrhoea, and dandruff in adults or "cradle cap" in infants. Signs and symptoms like yellow, oily, scaly patches on the scalp, face, ears, and other parts of the body, white flakes, intense itching and more occur.

Nummular eczema

Round, irritated, isolated patches occur on the arms and lower legs. Signs and symptoms like crust, scales, flakes and itching occur.

Lichen simplex chronicus

This is also known as localized neurodermatitis. It occurs due to continuous rubbing and scratching of the skin. Sensitivity or irritation of the skin leads to continuous itching and scratching. Signs and symptoms like scratch marks, thickened plaques on the neck, shins, wrists, or forearms, etc., occur. It improves when the patient stops itching and scratching.

Stasis dermatitis

This is a skin irritation found on the lower legs due to circulatory problems of the leg veins. It may occur with varicose veins. Signs and symptoms like dark, light brown or purplish-red pigmentation occur.

Dyshidrotic eczema

This is irritated skin commonly seen on the palms of the hands and soles of the feet. It is sometimes described as a "tapioca pudding" type of rash on the palms. Signs and symptoms like deep-seated blisters, itching and burning occur.

Xerotic eczema

This is a dry skin condition that occurs in elderly people. The lesions are commonly found on the lower legs.

Chapter 3: Causes of Atopic Dermatitis

The exact cause of Atopic Dermatitis is not known. The disease may be caused by genetic factors, surrounding environmental factors or a hyperactive immune system. Atopic Dermatitis is not an allergic reaction to any allergen or irritant. It is a chronic inflammatory condition of the skin where the skin remains chronically itchy. Hay fever and asthma are commonly related with Atopic Dermatitis, but they are not the cause of it. In many infants, Atopic Dermatitis resolves with age but they may develop hay fever or asthma in adulthood. Weakened immunity predisposes people to Atopic Dermatitis, and hence it is commonly found in infants who possess low immunity. Immunocompromised persons develop various skin diseases like fungal disease on their feet, staphylococcus, streptococcus boils on the skin, herpes simplex infection on the lips, etc., along with Atopic Dermatitis.

More than one gene is involved in the development of Atopic Dermatitis. If other atopic diseases like allergic rhinitis, asthma, etc., are found in a family, then the children have the risk of developing Atopic Dermatitis. The children are at more risk of developing the disease when both the parents are affected with any atopic disease.

Moreover, mutation in the gene involved in the production of filaggrin protein also predisposes one to the development of Atopic Dermatitis. The filaggrin protein is found in the epidermis of the skin and works at maintaining the protective skin barrier. The mutation in the gene alters the ability of filaggrin to protect the skin from various allergens, irritants and microorganisms. Thus the person has an increased risk of developing Atopic Dermatitis and other skin diseases.

1. Is Atopic Dermatitis Contagious or Spread by Touch and Close Contact?

Atopic Dermatitis is not contagious. Touch, kissing, shaking hands, eating with an affected person, etc, do not spread it. Remaining in close contact with individuals with Atopic Dermatitis does not harm healthy individuals. Precautions must be taken only when Atopic Dermatitis gets infected with staphylococcus, streptococcus and other bacteria, the herpes virus, yeasts and fungal infections. Secondary active infections can develop, which are highly contagious and spread through skin contact.

2. Who is Commonly Affected by Atopic Dermatitis?

Commonly, infants and young children are affected by Atopic Dermatitis, but it can occur in adults and elderly people too. The disease may appear and then disappear in the affected individual.

In a majority of patients there are periods of exacerbations or flare-ups where signs and symptoms are worse and the suffering of the patient increases, which is then followed by periods of remission where the signs and symptoms improve and the suffering is reduced. The skin clears up and seems as if there is no disease. As children grow older, complete clearance of the skin may be seen, but dryness and irritation of the skin may sometimes persist.

3. What are the Factors that Aggravate Atopic Dermatitis?

Various factors and conditions are present in the surrounding environment that can aggravate the signs and the symptoms of Atopic Dermatitis. These factors are both natural and artificial. Some of these factors are unavoidable as they are naturally present, but the patient can avoid some. Common aggravating factors include:

1) Dry skin with no moisture,

2) Sudden change in atmospheric temperature,

3) The low humidity conditions in bitter winter or cold weather,

4) Artificial cooling with air conditioners in hot weather (sudden change of temperature as it is hot outdoors and cold indoors),

5) The use of harsh, synthetic, rough, woolen and leather clothes,

6) The use of tight fitting clothes that don't allow the skin to breath and cause perspiration,

7) The use of harsh, highly perfumed soaps and detergents,

8) Continuous wetting of hands,

9) Frequent hand washing and face washing,

10) Excessive use of low quality cosmetics on the face and body,

11) Excessive use of alcoholic deodorants that irritate the skin,

12) Severe exercise which causes excessive perspiration on the body (perspiration aggravates itching),

13) The habit of exercising outdoors under direct exposure of harsh sunrays,

14) Working in industries where harsh synthetic chemicals are used,

15) Remaining underneath warm blankets for hours,

16) Taking a hot shower or bath and then suddenly moving in cold air,

17) Entering into a warm room after being in cold air,

18) Remaining unprotected in bitter winters,

and others.

All these factors have the common effect of triggering and aggravating the itch-scratch cycle. These factors also aggravate the overactive immune system of Atopic Dermatitis patients. Inflammation of the skin is increased, which leads to swelling, redness and dryness. The patient scratches repeatedly, which leads to breakage of the skin and the protective barrier of the skin is damaged. Harmful microorganisms set in and further deterioration of the skin condition occurs.

The mental status of the affected individual may also aggravate Atopic Dermatitis. Excessive sadness or happiness, nervous breakdown, mood swings, abnormal behavior, excessive cosmetic consciousness, obsessive-compulsive disorder, etc., have an effect on the skin condition of the patient. These emotional changes may cause the disease to flare up. In the case of an abnormal mental status, the patient does not have enough alertness to resist the itching and scratching. Conscious efforts are needed by the patient to avoid itching. Obsessive-compulsive disorder (OCD) patients may have a habit of frequent washing of their hands. They always feel that their hands are dirty and they cannot resist wetting them. The patients may use harsh soaps, which will aggravate Atopic Dermatitis.

A habit of frequent face washing is also commonly found in obsessive-compulsive disorder patients. This can aggravate Atopic Dermatitis. An OCD patient may even have a peculiar habit of scratching the whole body or particular body part even when an itch is not present. They simply cannot resist scratching. Continuous scratching may lead to a flare-up of underlying dormant Atopic Dermatitis.

A patient with Atopic Dermatitis may become irritated, agitated, restless and inattentive due to continuous itching and scratching. He or she may not be able to concentrate on work. Performance at home, work or school may be hampered.

In a broader context, these aggravating factors can be divided into two categories; irritants and allergens.

4. What are the Aggravating Skin Irritants of Atopic Dermatitis?

Irritants have a direct effect on the extremely sensitive skin of the Atopic Dermatitis patient. Irritants, when used for very long time and in high concentrations have a harmful effect on the skin. They may either flare up in the periodic cycle of the disease or may aggravate the ongoing disease phase. In some cases the irritants may prevent the cure of the patient. Correct diagnosis and the best possible treatment do not improve the skin condition of the patient because of the continuous exposure to the irritants. The skin becomes red, swollen, itchy, and may burn severely. Patients and their families need to identify what substances and irritants have a bad effect on the skin. They learn to identify this after frequent exposure to irritants and the subsequent bad effect. Various irritants have different effects on the skin. They may be mild to severe. For example, wearing woolen, leather or synthetic clothes may severely affect some patients of Atopic Dermatitis and some may have a milder effect. Rough and tight-fitting clothes may cause irritation, inflammation, and perspiration in some patients, while some others may be affected with rough, loose fitting clothes.

A few patients may be affected by perfumed soaps and detergents that cause drying and itching, while some patients are not affected at all by the use of soaps and detergents. Low quality perfumes, deodorants and cosmetics generally affect all Atopic Dermatitis patients to varying degrees. A few Atopic Dermatitis patients are so sensitive to these deodorants and cosmetics that they are not able to use them at all. Bathing in the excessively chlorinated water of a swimming pool may aggravate excessive itching. Exposure to solvents, oil, factory chemicals, dust or sand leads to triggering of the "itch-scratch cycle."

Cigarette smoking, both active and passive, badly affects Atopic Dermatitis on the face and eyes. Housewives, females working in offices, infants, etc., are usually exposed to passive smoking. Skin gets irritated as the smoke comes in contact with the skin.

Use of narcotics and other forms of tobacco may also aggravate Atopic Dermatitis.

Children tend to play in dust, mud, sand and dirty surroundings. Hence they come into close contact with these irritants, which stay on their bodies for long periods of time. Lesions of the disease are contaminated with the bacteria and spores present in the dirt and mud. Hence there is a high risk of infection, which damages the skin to a great extent. Housewives and maids come into close contact with dust while cleaning the house and offices. They may be affected with dust, debris and dust mites, which irritate the skin and induce itching.

Fur and the hairs of pet animals are common irritants, which many patients of Atopic Dermatitis are unaware of. Infants, children and adults commonly play and spend time with pets, which may irritate the hypersensitive skin of the Atopic Dermatitis patient and leads to severe itching and scratching. Pet animals lick the skin of the patient, which may further deteriorate the disease, as the saliva of pets is highly irritable for the skin. Walking and playing in gardens where the person is exposed to pollens, flowers, grass, etc., may also irritate the skin.

Those Atopic Dermatitis patients who have the hobby of gardening do not tend to improve, as close contact with pollens and flowers serves as a maintaining cause of the disease. (Maintaining causes are those causes that maintain the progress of the disease and do not allow improvement even though the best treatment is employed).

Common Irritants are summarised below:

1) Woolen, leather or synthetic clothes

2) Harsh soaps and washing detergents

3) Low quality perfumes and deodorants

4) Low quality cosmetics

5) Irritants such as chlorine, industrial oil, or solvents

6) Dust, sand or debris

7) Dust mites

8) Cigarette smoke

9) Animal fur or dander (dander are small particles that are found on animal skin, especially in cats and dogs)

10) Flowers or pollens

5. What are Allergens that Aggravate Atopic Dermatitis?

Allergens or allergic substances may be found in foods, plants, or animals. Inflammation sets in as a result of contact with allergens. Allergens activate the hyperactive immune system of a person. Irritation and inflammation can occur even when the person comes into minimal contact with the allergen. Allergic reactions occur even when a hypersensitive person comes into contact with the allergen for a very short period of time. Animal hair, fur, and dander act as irritants as well as allergens.

Plants that secrete waxy materials or have strong fragrances may serve as allergens for a sensitive patient and cause severe itching. Pollens, especially in winter weather, are highly allergic. People residing around farms and gardens are prone to developing allergic Atopic Dermatitis due to contact with pollens. These pollens, animal hairs and fur activate the inflammatory cells of the body. These cells release chemicals that cause swelling, redness, and itching. The patient scratches the skin severely and bleeding may occur, which may further worsen inflammation.

What are Aeroallergens?

Aeroallergens are those allergens that are present in the air. Aeroallergens initiate allergic reactions and aggravate Atopic Dermatitis. Common aeroallergens include minute dust particles, dust mites, pollens, molds, and dander. The most irritating aeroallergen that initiates and aggravates Atopic Dermatitis is the house dust mite. Housewives and maids are the common victims of house dust mites. They worsen itching and scratching of Atopic Dermatitis.

There are mixed opinions about the role of aeroallergens in initiating and aggravating Atopic Dermatitis. Some researchers and doctors are in flavor of the theory that aeroallergens are the major contributing factors in aggravating Atopic Dermatitis. Some researchers and doctors do not agree with this theory and firmly believe that aeroallergens have no role in initiating or worsening Atopic Dermatitis. They consider them least important.

Reliable tests determining the role of aeroallergens and confirming particular aeroallergens as causative and aggravating factors in Atopic Dermatitis are not yet available. In conditions where the treating allergist or dermatologist suspects that an aeroallergen is enhancing the signs and the symptoms of the patient and is becoming a hindrance in the way of cure or relieving symptoms, they may advise the patient to reduce exposure to the aeroallergens as much as possible. Complete avoidance of aeroallergens is not practically possible, since they are abundantly found in the surrounding air.

Certain methods or practices can be adopted that can reduce exposure. For example, the house dust mite can be restricted in houses by using dust-proof covers for encasing mattresses and pillows. They do not allow dust mites to accumulate on pillows and mattresses. Clothes, bed sheets, and carpets must be washed at shorter intervals so that dust and dirt does not accumulate on them. Hot water is preferred for washing. Dirty clothes should not be worn. Efforts should be made to keep the house and office clean where the patient spends the most time. Regular cleaning must be done. Precautions must be taken while cleaning. Gloves and scarves must be used while cleaning, and direct contact with dirty material should be avoided.

Many treating dermatologists advise the patients of Atopic Dermatitis not to keep pet animals at home. If they still want to keep pets, precautions must be taken while coming in contact with animals. Soft gloves can be used while handling them. Pets must be kept hygienically, so daily bathing and combing of hairs and furs of the pet must be done.

Chapter 4: Does Food Cause Atopic Dermatitis?

Sensitivity to various foods and eating habits are usually not related to Atopic Dermatitis. Several research studies are ongoing to find a relation between food and the disease. However, certain foods and food preservatives are highly allergenic. They may induce allergic inflammation and worsen Atopic Dermatitis. Food allergens commonly affect infants and children having Atopic Dermatitis as they are more sensitive to food allergens compared to adults. Common allergic reactions to food include urticaria (red or white hives on the skin), gastric disturbances like nausea, vomiting, diarrhea, respiratory tract symptoms like congestion, sneezing, runny nose, wheezing, coughing, etc., lacrimation from eyes (tears from eyes), swelling of the face and eyes, etc. The common food substances that cause allergy include eggs, peanuts, peanut butter, milk and milk products, fish, soya milk and soya products, wheat, meat and more.

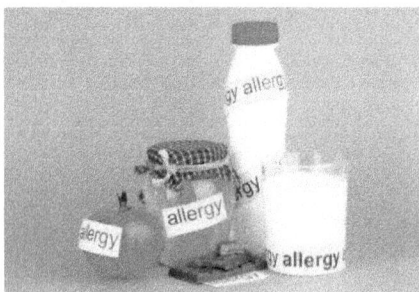

A few studies advise women to avoid these allergic foods during pregnancy, especially those women who have a family history of atopic diseases. They must also avoid these allergic substances while breastfeeding the infants. These studies are yet not clearly established, but still-pregnant and nursing women must take these precautions to prevent Atopic Dermatitis.

Breastfeeding must be encouraged; as many studies conducted by researchers and doctors flavor that breastfeeding the infant for at least six months provides protection to the infant against various allergies, including Atopic Dermatitis. Breast milk contains antibodies (those substances in the body that fight against harmful substances), and protective proteins and vitamins, which are necessary for withstanding allergens and infections.

Many researchers promote the fact that excessive protection should not be given to infants and children. Theories suggest that infants and children must be allowed to live and play freely in the open environment. All types of food including allergic foods must be given. Exposure to the natural environment and allergic foods in early months and years builds up the natural immunity of the person. This renders the person safe against common, natural allergic substances. His or her body becomes capable of fighting against various environmental contaminants. This natural immunity helps in preventing Atopic Dermatitis in infants and children.

In cases of suspected food allergy, the person must write down all the foods he or she eats daily. After writing down the food substances, a list of the food must be made which triggered allergic reactions of any kind. It may not be easy for the person to identify the food allergen, but still efforts must be made.

The help of an allergist (an expert in treating allergy) may be used by the person to identify the food allergen. Allergists keenly observe the food pattern of the person and the type of allergic reaction evoked. After identifying the suspected food, it may be stopped for two weeks, and if an improvement in the allergic reaction is noted, it is again consumed gradually after two weeks under the supervision of the allergist. This kind of trial for every suspected food must be done for two weeks. If the food being tested causes symptoms on reintroduction, it is confirmed that the person is allergic to that particular food. If no symptoms occur after reintroduction, it can be considered that person is not allergic to that particular food. A two-week trial of every food is sufficient for identifying a food allergen.

Complete restriction of the allergic food must be immediately practiced. A careful medical, family and personal history of the person must be taken. A repeat trial of stopping the suspected allergic food for two weeks and its reintroduction must be done for confirmation. If the history and the trial confirm the food allergy and the aggravation of Atopic Dermatitis, restriction must be made and the person may stop eating the allergic food substance.

After stopping the food, it is incumbent upon the person, family members and the treating physician to decide how much improvement is actually seen in signs and symptoms of the Atopic Dermatitis. If visible improvement is not seen and felt by the person, reconsideration of the decision to stop the food allergen must be done. Restricting the food or changing diet may not benefit every Atopic Dermatitis patient.

Moreover, restricting and stopping the food may be difficult for many people. They may feel stress in stopping the food. This emotional imbalance may worsen the condition instead of improve it. Financial losses may be encountered by family members when commonly available foods are stopped and special foods are advised.

Nutritional problems may be encountered in infants, children and adults on stopping allergic foods since many people may be allergic to foods that are highly nutritious like eggs, meat, fish, soya milk, etc. It may happen that the person may be left with only a few foods to eat, which can lead to severe malnutrition. Malnutrition is common in children due to protein, vitamin and mineral deficiency, which may be aggravated by food restriction. Careful guidance by the allergist and nutritionist is needed to prevent nutritional problems. Hence, identifying the food allergen, stopping the food, and restarting the food must all be done under the strict observation of an expert allergist, nutritionist and dermatologist.

Chapter 5: How Did I Develop the Problem?

Atopic Dermatitis usually has an early onset of signs and symptoms. It may start as early as two months of age. Dry skin and patchy rashes are found around the lips, cheeks, chin, hands and feet. Nipple eczema may occur. The palms may have more creases and scaling. Various allergy tests like the prick test, food allergy test, etc., are positive. Serum IgE levels are high and the skin has a tendency to get repeated infections.

(Note - Detailed description of allergy tests and serum IgE levels is discussed in Chapter 6.)

1. What are the Signs and Symptoms of Atopic Dermatitis?

The lesions of Atopic Dermatitis are commonly found in adults and older children on the folds of the skin in front of the elbow, the back of the knees and around the mouth. In infants the lesions are seen on the chin, cheeks, scalp, extremities, diaper area, etc. Various types of symptoms are found in the disease. Every patient has a varied form of the disease. Mild Atopic Dermatitis affects a smaller zone of the body, whereas severe Atopic Dermatitis may be widespread and cover the whole body. Commonly found signs and symptoms include dryness, itching, scratching, rubbing, and redness of the skin. Itching is the first and the most prominent symptom of Atopic Dermatitis. Itching is usually followed by a rash that may appear and disappear. The rash may be acute or chronic in the patient. Some patients may constantly suffer from red patches all over the body for years. The rash is usually dry and flaky, but when the patient scratches, it becomes inflamed and may ooze. Fluid filled sores may be found in the acute stage, which ooze and crusts may form. In the sub-acute stage dry, red, itchy skin is found. In the chronic stage dry, thick and tough areas known as lichenification are found.

Infants of two months to two years old generally have oozing rashes on their cheeks and chin. The rashes become severe in the winter. Older children of two to eleven years pass through various stages of lesions. Oozing rashes turn into dry rashes. Oozing is generally not found in older children, and lichenfication commonly occurs. The lesions of Atopic Dermatitis are found more on sites such as the folds of the arms, front of the elbow, and back of the knees, wrists, face, and hands. Less common sites of affection are behind the ears, groin, and other parts of the body. Skin inflammation is worsened with progression of the disease. Patients with Atopic Dermatitis develop an "itch-scratch" cycle where severe itching leads to scratching and scratching again aggravates itching. The patient scratches it more and more severely and the skin inflammation worsens. Patients with Atopic Dermatitis are more sensitive to itching compared to other skin diseases. These patients need to scratch more severely and for longer periods of time to get relief from itching compared to other skin diseases.

Itching is severely aggravated during the night and sleep. The patient does not have consciousness to control the scratching. Other stimuli are also not present in the surroundings, which can divert the attention of the patient from itching and scratching. The patient unconsciously notices the itch more, and scratches it. Thus the "itch-scratch" cycle starts. Itching may be worse even during the evening since after returning home from the office or school, the individual does not have enough work or stimulus to distract the mind from the itching. Some patients develop an active immune system, which results in more active, red, scaly skin. Some patients develop lichenification where thick, leathery, dry skin occurs due to constant scratching. Lichenification occurs in the later stage of the disease. Lichenification indicates that the disease has progressed to a chronic stage. Lichenification appears after rashes fade away. Some patients develop papules, blisters and tiny raised bumps on the skin. They scratch the papule severely, which opens it. The papule may ooze and becomes crusty. Furthermore, the skin gets infected. The skin of the Atopic Dermatitis patient is usually dry and hence the risk of developing irritant contact dermatitis is always high.

2. Various skin features of Atopic Dermatitis.

The skin features of Atopic Dermatitis are:

1) L i c h e n i f i c a t i o n : The skin becomes thick, leathery, hard and dry due to continuous itching and scratching.

2) Lichen simplex: A thick patch develops on the skin, which is raised. It occurs due to constant rubbing and scratching of the patch.

3) Papules: These are tiny, raised bumps that break due to scratching. They may ooze and become crusty. Infection sets in due to open skin.

4) Ichthyosis: Dry, scaly skin is found, commonly on the lower limbs, especially the legs and shins. The lesions are rectangular in shape.

5) Keratosis pilaris: Tiny, uneven, rough bumps with coiled hair underneath develop on the face, upper arms, and thighs. They look like gooseflesh or chicken skin.

6) Hyper linear palms: Skin on the palms develops many more folds and creases than normally found.

7) Urticaria: Red and white raised hives develop on the skin, which is accompanied by severe itching. Fever may be found along with it. It develops after exposure to an irritating allergen, allergic food, exercise, very cold and hot weather. It may indicate the beginning of a flare-up phase of the disease.

8) Cheilitis: This is the inflamed skin of the lips and surrounding areas.

9) Atopic pleat (Dennie-Morgan fold): This is an extra fold of skin that develops under the eye as an effect of Atopic Dermatitis around the eyes.

10) Dark circles under the eyes: They may occur due to irritation of the skin due to irritants and allergens.

11) Hyperpigmented eyelids: Dark brown and black-pigmented eyelids occur due to inflammation of the eyelids and hay fever.

12) Prurigo nodules: This is also known as "picker's warts." They are small, thick bumps of skin due to repeated scratching and rubbing at the same skin area. They are actually not real warts.

3. How does Atopic Dermatitis Affect the Face?

Atopic Dermatitis commonly affects the skin around the eyes. Infants are more affected on the face. In infants, saliva dribbles from the mouth, which irritates the affected skin. Infants unknowingly touch the face frequently and their contact with external irritable stimuli is also high, which aggravates the disease.

Severe itching and scratching is found on the eyelids, the eyebrows, and the lashes. The appearance of the skin around the eyes is changed. An atopic pleat or Dennie-Morgan fold, which is an extra fold of skin under eye, develops. Hyperpigmented eyelids (dark blackish, brown pigmentation of skin on the eyelids) may develop due to severe inflammation of the eyelids and hay fever. Swollen, patchy eyelids, eyebrows and eyelashes may occur due to irritation and inflammation of the skin caused by scratching and rubbing.

Skin with no moisture on the face is found. Dryness is caused in the epidermis as few patients with Atopic Dermatitis possess a defective genetic trait where a protein called fillagrin, which is very essential for retaining moisture and preventing dryness in the epidermis, is not found. Due to moisture loss, the skin loses its protective ability and becomes susceptible to harmful and irritable agents. Severe dryness leads to growth of pathogens like staphylococcus, streptococcus bacteria, virus and fungi, which lead to skin infections like boils, blisters, warts, herpes simplex on the lips, back, and molluscum contagiosum.

4. What are the Stages of Atopic Dermatitis?

Every child with Atopic Dermatitis may have different symptoms. The onset, duration and severity of the disease vary in every child. Infants are usually affected with Atopic Dermatitis at around 1 ½ to 3 months of age. In the beginning, the disease commonly appears as a rash and a patch on the face. The rash is usually around the cheeks and the chin. Then as the disease further progresses, the skin becomes red, scaly and inflamed, which may ooze. Infection sets in due to severe scratching and rubbing, which breaks the protective barrier of the skin and the skin is exposed to harmful environmental pathogens.

As the infants grow the areas such as the knees and elbows also get affected and the disease may spread to distal limbs and throughout the body. Severe itching leads to irritability and the infants become restless, irritable, anxious, agitated and uncomfortable in any given surrounding. Infants usually improve around four to five months of age but they may suffer from dry skin or hand eczema in adulthood. In slightly older babies the rash usually occurs at the back of the knees, on the elbows, on the sides of the neck, wrists, ankles, and hands. Papules are found along with rashes on these sites. The papules are hard, scaly, crusty and itchy. Inflammation of the skin on the lips and surrounding areas is found. The child is tempted to constantly lick and prick the lips and surrounding areas. This leads to painful cracks on sensitive skin of lips, which may even bleed. The disease may be localized to any one part of the body or may be generalized.

Advanced and well-spread Atopic Dermatitis hampers the normal growth of the child in terms of height. The affected child may be shorter in height in comparison to a child without Atopic Dermatitis. The disease has a cyclical tendency where periods of flare and periods of remission are seen. The affected child may have a symptom-free stage for months or even years. A majority of children have complete remission of the disease when they enter into adolescence and puberty.

The disease usually does not begin in the later years of life. However, those adults who have had the disease when they were very young may experience a sudden flare-up of signs and symptoms. Usually adults and children have a similar course of the disease. The disease may be localized to one area or may spread throughout the body. The disease may be limited to only the hands or feet, which become severely dry, itchy, red, and cracked. A rash around the nipples may also occur. Cataracts may also develop. Adults suffer from disturbed sleep due to night aggravation of the itching and scratching. The work quality of adults is affected due to attention only to the itching and not in work.

Patients with Atopic Dermatitis are at a high risk of developing irritant contact dermatitis, which develops due to contact with irritants like cement, oil, harsh chemicals like soda bicarbonate, hydrochloric acid; solvents, etc., used in industries. Individuals working in kitchens or doing washing work like maids need to wet and wash their hands frequently, hence they have increased their risk of developing irritant contact dermatitis.

Generalized symptoms are easy to treat, but localized symptoms on any one site are difficult to treat since people do not narrate the symptoms completely to the treating physician due their ignorance or embarrassment. Eye examinations are recommended regularly since patients with Atopic Dermatitis may easily ignore a developing cataract, which does not show early symptoms. Medications are given for a very long time to treat symptoms and hence they may cause complications and drug disease.

5. What are the Complications of Atopic Dermatitis?
The most common complication of Atopic Dermatitis is altered

skin color. The area on which skin lesions are found may become lighter or darker in color in comparison to the normal skin tone. The tone of the skin changes due to constant scratching, rubbing and friction on the skin. The altered skin is commonly found on the face, hands, upper arms, shoulders, back, etc. The lighter or the darken patches gradually come back into normal skin tone after complete healing of the symptoms.

Secondary bacterial infections on the skin due to Staphylococcus, Streptococcus, S.Aureus, etc., cause fever, pain, malaise, boils, abscess, sores, etc.

The herpes simplex virus infects the Atopic Dermatitis lesions and causes eczema herpeticum. Rashes and blisters of the disease start oozing serum and blood. Fever develops and crusts form on the skin. Cold sores may develop, which take a long time to heal.

A secondary fungal infection like ring worm may occur, which can be dry or wet, along with continuous itching.

Permanent scars can develop on the skin due to severe scratching, rubbing and bleeding.

Local and systemic side effects can occur due to the long-term treatment of the disease. Topical corticosteroids may cause local side effects like petechial hemorrhage (small, red spots appear on the skin due to hemorrhage), thin skin, atrophy of skin, severe acne, stretch marks etc. Systemic side effects like growth failure in children, weak bones, etc., may occur. Calcineurine inhibitors may cause burning, irritation and skin cancer.

Children may develop fearfulness, shyness, dependency, mood changes, irritability and tiredness due to stress and anxiety associated with the disease. Children and adults both may loose sleep due to night aggravation of disease. Loss of sleep can badly affect health. Moreover, the habit of waking at night may even continue after the lesions have cleared up. Patients may require sleeping pills for getting good sleep.

6. What is the prognosis of Atopic Dermatitis?

The prognosis of Atopic Dermatitis is favorable. The disease can be managed effectively if proper treatment and care is taken. The prognosis is favorable since the majority of children improve by adolescence. Prognosis is unfavorable when the disease develops at a young age, in immunocompromised patients like HIV positive or cancer patients, in severe, widespread disease, asthma, hay fever, urticarial, etc., along with Atopic Dermatitis, family history, etc.

The signs and the symptoms of Atopic Dermatitis are difficult to treat and they take a long time to heal. The disease may relapse often. Yet, the patients of Atopic Dermatitis can live a healthy life. Support from family and surrounding people help the patient to live a normal life with social wellbeing. The families of the patient can also live stress free if they follow the prescribed treatment and understand the disease thoroughly. In acute flare-ups, the physician should be contacted immediately, and required treatment must be completed for a favorable prognosis.

For long-term management of Atopic Dermatitis, an allergist and a dermatologist should be regularly visited. Allergists help in managing allergies. They can determine the allergen and can teach the patient how to stay away from it, which becomes very helpful for long-term management of the disease. A dermatologist can regularly monitor and examine the skin. Timely checkups by a dermatologist can help to immediately start the treatment if any alarming signs and symptoms of a flare-up are found. Flare-ups and relapses can be aborted very quickly this way. This helps in long-term management of the disease.

7. Does Atopic Dermatitis have any effect on the quality of life?

No, Atopic Dermatitis does not have any significant effect on the quality of life. Atopic Dermatitis causes lesions all over the body or on exposed parts of the body like the face, hands, legs, neck etc. The lesions may range from mild, moderate or severe. In some patients these lesions may be so mild that they even may not be visible. Moderate or severe lesions may be widespread and the patient may find them embarrassing. Patients find themselves ugly looking when the lesions are on the exposed parts of the body. Adults and children may have a feeling of inferiority that they are not beautiful. But despite the signs and symptoms caused by Atopic Dermatitis, it is possible for people suffering from the disorder to maintain a high quality of life. The disorder should not be given importance. Patients should very clearly understand the fact that Atopic Dermatitis is a very casual skin disorder found in a large number of people in the world. It has no effect on the quality of life and the patient need not feel strange or ashamed about it. Atopic Dermatitis is easily curable with little precautions. It does not have any effect on the life span of the patient. It does not cause any deep-seated disease in the body. It does not affect vital organs of the body like the heart, brain, lungs or kidney. It does not spread by touching, kissing, hanging out together, living together o r eating together. It does not even spread by having sexual relations with the affected person.

The treatment of Atopic Dermatitis is also very simple and easy to follow. In the initial phase, the patient is given only a soap-free cleanser and gentle moisturizer to use. The patient may easily adapt to the prescribed regimen and will be quickly relieved from the disease. In later stages, corticosteroids are given for external application along with a few oral medicines. The medicines are usually freely available and the patient will generally have to take it only once or twice a day. Hence, following the treatment plan is not very bothersome for the patient. The prescribed medicines and external applications usually do not cause any side effects. They are safe and well proved. These medicines and topical applications have no effect on quality of life. All that information is conveyed by the physician to the patient.

A comfortable communication level is set between the patient and physician, who very calmly explains to the patient that his or her disease is easily curable and she should not feel hesitant about asking any questions related to the disease. The physician may even demonstrate to the patient any procedure that needs to be followed correctly during the treatment regimen. For example, if the patient has the bad habit of scratching the lesions with his/her nails, the physician demonstrates to the patient that instead of nails, a gentle piece of cotton or soft material can be used for gently rubbing the lesions. The physician will educate the patient and family members about the disease in the simplest language. This will help the patient to better understand the disease. It may boost the confidence of the patient to know that the disease is very common and it has no effect on the quality of life.

Atopic Dermatitis awareness programs are held by many physicians and dermatologists. Awareness programs are even held by non-government organizations, institutes, and forums that are working for the benefit of people suffering from the disease. A patient should attend these awareness programs as they provide the latest information about the disease and the treatments available. These awareness programs boost the confidence of patients and they start feeling better after attending them. Education programs are also held by many societies, schools, colleges, physician groups and governments. These educational programs are attended by patients, relatives and also those people who do not suffer from the disease. This helps to educate people and to get rid of the myths prevailing about Atopic Dermatitis in society. These education and awareness programs allow the patient to interact with people having similar complaints. By this way, they will also learn new information about the disease, which will also relieve some of the stress.

A good partnership between patient, physician and family will greatly benefit and improve the quality of life of the patient. Support from friends and family members are of great importance during treatment. Encouragement from friends and family members is required in following the daily skin care regimen, taking timely medication and going for regular check-ups. All these points are the key to improving the patient's quality of life.

Adults may be able to tackle the problems related to Atopic Dermatitis easily. They face fewer problems in managing the frustration related to the disease, but infants and children find it extremely difficult to manage Atopic Dermatitis and issues related to it. Along with infants and children, the parents, family members and friends are all affected. Children feel extremely frustrated due to the severe itching and burning associated with the disease. Itching makes them restless, agitated and angry. They may become very demanding and moody. Slightly older children may be taught how to resist itching, but when infants are affected, they cannot be taught, which leads to a miserable condition. They are not able to resist itching and even cannot express complaints.

Parents and guardians of the babies must be very patient and cooperative with them. Even after many efforts, children may not be able to keep from itching, scratching and rubbing. Additional support must be given by the parents in managing the stress associated with the disease. Parents should help children learn how to gently rub the skin when itching arises and how to distract their attention towards other activities when the itch arises. Children may not learn this easily, but the parents should make genuine, repeated efforts to teach them. They must be taught activities in which the hands remain busy.

For example, playing piano, drawing pictures, painting on a canvas, working on computers, etc. In these activities, the hands remain busy and children will be distracted from itching. In infants, these activities may not be possible. In the case of infants, parents should continuously remain with them and should distract them when they are tempted to scratch. Parents can distract the infant by whistling, by making some noise, by showing some toys, by lifting up the child, by playing with fingers, etc. Soft baby gloves are also available on the market, which can be used so that babies do not scratch the lesions with fingernails.

Children must be encouraged to play outdoors with their friends and be involved in outdoor hobbies. Parents should not confine children inside the house. Being confined in the house can discourage the child. Children should be sent to school regularly, although it may be difficult for them to manage at school due to itching and the appearance of lesions. Parents should make the children understand that they are not different from others. The lesions are very common and they will be soon relieved.

Parents can even talk to the schoolteacher, school attendants and other caretakers about the lesions so that they can help the children when they are at school or in other care settings. Schoolteachers and parents should take special care that the social relationship of the child is not hampered. If any block or stigma develops in the early years, children may suffer from it throughout their life. For example, a child may feel shy about meeting friends or playing with them due to their skin problems. He or she may become introverted and cling to the mother.

If this behavior is not attended to, and the child is not encouraged to play outdoors and meet other people, then he/she may suffer from major depression and an inferiority complex later on in adolescence and adulthood. Parents should be aware of any emotional or social stress due to the appearance of the child. Parents should clearly understand that disfigurement caused by the lesions of Atopic Dermatitis is not permanent. It will be relieved with proper care. Pessimistic behavior of parents can badly affect the quality of their children's lives.

Adults having Atopic Dermatitis should follow their skin care regimen daily. This will help them in improving their quality of life. Efforts should be made to perform the skin care regimen daily. Easy skin care regimens can be developed by the physician and the patient that can be followed every day in any circumstance and for any skin condition. It should be kept in mind that the skin care regimen should not be stopped when the skin has improved significantly and also when the skin has deteriorated a lot. It should be continued throughout the year. A daily skin care regimen will prevent a flare-up phase of the disease from occurring. And even if a flare-up phase occurs, it will be controlled, with tolerable signs and symptoms.

Quality of life can be greatly improved when the person is aware all the time about the disease. Ignorance can greatly damage the skin and the patient's perceptions. As soon as symptoms of a flare-up phase appear, the patient should immediately contact the physician. There should be no delay in seeking treatment. Many patients believe that taking the treatment will harm them instead of benefitting them. In this case, they may never seek medical advice and their disease will go on deteriorating. Some patients may rely only on alternative therapies and home treatments. This should not be done. A patient can take alternative therapies, which are universally accepted and have shown good improvement, along with main conventional treatment. Too many experiments on the skin should not be done. Every new thing suggested by anyone should not be tried. One should think over and research the idea before using it. Haphazardly trying everything will result in nothing. All this ignorance can harm the patient and can hamper his/her quality of life.

Stress and anxiety can greatly affect the quality of life. Stress management and relaxation techniques can be very helpful in improving quality of life. Patients should be involved in activities they are most interested in. These include: 1) listening to music, 2) reading interesting books, 3) participating in sports activities, 4) learning new skills, 5) developing new hobbies, 6) doing in creative writing, 7) attending nature camps where one remains close to nature, 8) pursuing higher studies, 9) participating in social gatherings, 10) working for the needy, 11) working with organizations that are involved in social activities, 12) helping family members around the house, 13) cooking, 14) exercising, 15) meditation, 16) yoga, etc., may all be very helpful for the patient in relieving stress.

Overworking also should not be done. Overworking can lead to stress and a flare-up of the disease. Patients should take timely breaks from work. Stress due to the disease condition also needs to be managed. If a patient is not able to manage by him or herself, then he/she should seek help from family members and friends. Talking and opening up about the stress will help greatly to relieve it. Patients can even seek help of the treating physician or a psychologist.

Counseling taken from an expert psychologist can be more beneficial, as it is more scientific. Patients may open up more with an unknown psychologist in comparison to known family members. A psychologist can make the patient thoroughly understand that the stress is only increasing his/her complaints. Short-term psychotherapy can be very helpful with the depression and anxiety that may occur due to the disease. A psychologist may even prescribe mild anxiolytic drugs (those drugs which relieve anxiety) and sleeping pills in severe cases where psychotherapy is not sufficient. Sleeping pills help the patient to get a sound sleep. The sleep of Atopic Dermatitis patients is usually disturbed due to night aggravation. Sound sleep will freshen up the patient the next day and attention to itching will also be reduced at night. The psychologist will always take care that these pills do not become habit forming for the patient, who should not use them for a very long time and should always take them in the prescribed dose under the strict supervision of the psychologist. Many Atopic Dermatitis patients suffer from minor depression due to their appearance and severe itching that persists all the time. Itching can become a cause of embarrassment at work and in public places. Patients cannot control the itching even though they try hard at doing so.

Patients feel that they are the subjects of jokes and that people are laughing at them. This might not be true and people may not have even noticed the person or the habit of itching. But constant anxiety about itching and the fear that someone will notice them and laugh at them causes minor depression in some patients with Atopic Dermatitis. These patients require extra support from family members and friends. Psychotherapy and sleeping pills are helpful in relieving depression.

Certain organizations and groups can also be helpful to these patients. These organizations provide a common platform for all Atopic Dermatitis patients to meet each other. When patients having similar complaints meet each other, they can interact with each other and exchange thoughts and ideas about the disease. New things can be learned about how to overcome the disease and the problems associated with it. The experience of other people who have suffered from Atopic Dermatitis and have overcome it can be very useful for other patients. Hence support from family members, friends, the physician, groups and organizations working for Atopic Dermatitis can be very beneficial. When all these people come together and make a combined effort, patients surely get relief from the problems.

Patients should identify and make a record about the time itching is likely to occur. They should maintain a diary noting the time or the situation when the itch is aggravated. After repeated efforts of this kind, patients may be able to find out the situation or time when the itch becomes severe. For example, the patient may find that the itch is aggravated in the evening or at night time, during heavy perspiration, after exposure to the sun, when staying idle, while coming into contact with certain plants or pets, etc. This may help him/her to stay away from these factors so that itching and scratching can be prevented. He/she should always try to remain occupied in some type of work. Remaining idle will draw attention to the itch. The patient must engage in structured activity where the hands do not remain free, so the time he/she is doing some quality work is not wasted in itching. The mind and the energy of the person must be channeled into work. For example, the patient can develop an interest in computer work where the hands are used continuously or in piano playing where the fingers remain busy, etc. This will gradually help in controlling the itch-scratch cycle and it may disappear with time.

A patient may even need to change his/her profession if the maintaining cause or triggering factor of Atopic Dermatitis is involved with the profession. For example, if a patient is an auto mechanic or a worker in an industry where he/she is continuously exposed to oil, chemicals, irritants, etc., then they will need to either leave the job or get transferred into another department. Another example is a woman with Atopic Dermatitis on the hands who is serving as a maid or a cook where she will need to wash her hands repeatedly. She may need to change her work, as constant wetting of the hands will not allow the lesions of Atopic Dermatitis to heal.

The help of an occupational counselor can be useful. This advisor will be able to counsel the patient to leave the job or change the type of profession. A patient may find this very troublesome, since leaving the job or changing the profession is not mentally and financially comfortable for anyone. Patients are made to understand the fact that their health is more important in comparison to the profession. Changing the profession can be done with few difficulties, but living with lesions that are increasing due to the profession may ultimately harm the patient more. Patients may suffer from emotional setback, as they may not be able to accept the change easily. They may not even be able to find new work or adapt to new work. This may again cause emotional issues, which may trigger another episode of Atopic Dermatitis. To prevent such emotional issues, the help of occupational counselors, family members and the physician can be very useful.

Patients are sometimes involved in such hobbies that may flare up Atopic Dermatitis. Patients may even not know about this or if they know, they may not be giving importance to it. For example, a patient has the hobby of beach volleyball hence he/she will often visit the beach in the open sun. They will play under the harsh sun and will come into contact with salty water for a long time. Beach sand will constantly touch the skin. Many times the patient forgets to apply sun block or he/she may apply low quality sun block. They will stay for a long time under the sun and will perspire a lot. All these factors will combine together and irritate the skin and the "itch-scratch" cycle will begin. Lesions will not heal even after good treatment. Hence many times a patient will have to give up the hobby. It depends upon the physician to advise the patient whether to give up the hobby permanently or temporarily until the lesions heal. The physician usually decides this after complete examination of the lesions and determining the role of the hobby in increasing the lesions.

Giving up the hobby permanently or even temporarily can become difficult for the patient since hobbies are the activities the person is most interested in. Family members should extend extra support to the patient during this phase. Family members should encourage the patient to develop a new hobby and take interest in that. Adults may be able to adopt new hobbies, but children may face great difficulties in doing so. If adults or children are not able to cope with the altered situation, then the help of hobby developers can be taken. They can easily introduce new hobbies to adults and children.

Chapter 6: Ways of Diagnosing Atopic Dermatitis

1. How to diagnose Atopic Dermatitis?

Examination of the patient:

Physical examination, visual inspection and observation of the skin are done by a physician or dermatologist to diagnose Atopic Dermatitis. A thorough personal and family history of the patient is required to be taken. History of rashes, hay fever (seasonal allergies) and asthma is inquired about as they may accompany Atopic Dermatitis.

Various tests done for diagnosis of Atopic Dermatitis are as follows:

1) Skin swab test
2) Blood test
3) Biopsy test
4) Allergy test- a) Skin allergy test b) Blood allergy test c) Food allergy test

Skin swab test

A skin swab test is done when infection with bacteria like staphylococcus and streptococcus is suspected. In this test, a long cotton tip applicator is used. It is rolled over the skin where the bacterial infection is suspected and it is sent to a laboratory for culture and examination. This test is helpful in diagnosis of secondary bacterial infection, which worsens and complicates the skin condition of the patient.

Blood test

Patients with severe atopic disease are advised to go for a blood test. Complete blood count is advised. A patient usually has an increased number of eosinophils (a type of white blood cells), which release antihistamines against allergens.

White blood cell count is also increased when the secondary bacterial infection with staphylococcus, streptococcus bacteria occurs. The cell count is increased as a result of the defensive mechanism of the body. WBC fights against the secondary infections.

Biopsy of skin

Biopsy of the skin means a skin sample from the affected area is taken and is sent to a laboratory for microscopic examination of tissues and cells. The skin sample is taken in required amount by expert dermatologist. This test is costly and is also not very useful in diagnosis of the disease. It is usually recommended when skin cancer is suspected along with Atopic Dermatitis.

Allergy tests

Allergy tests are done to find out the possible allergens that may trigger Atopic Dermatitis or may aggravate the present condition of the patient. A skin allergy test or a blood test is done. Usually it is preferable to do a skin test in comparison to a blood test since skin tests are cheap, accurate and rapid.

Skin tests

In the skin test the suspected allergen is exposed to the skin. It is placed on the skin and the skin is observed for response and reaction.

Usually three types of skin tests are done:

1) Skin prick test
2) Intradermal test

3) Skin patch test

Skin prick test: In this test an allergen solution is placed on the skin and the skin is scratched or pricked with a needle. Scratching and pricking allows the allergen to enter the skin. When the person is allergic to the introduced allergen, the red elevated wheal develops at the site of introduction of the allergen. The area becomes severely itchy.

The skin prick test is helpful in knowing the sensitivity of the person to the allergens like pollens, pet hair and dander, plants, trees, dust, feathers etc present in the surroundings. It can be helpful in knowing the allergies to foods like soya products, milk products, shellfish, nuts, sour items, eggs etc.

Intradermal test: This test is done in those individuals in whom the skin prick test turns out to be negative but there still is suspicion of allergic reaction by that particular allergen for which the skin prick test was performed. In this test a solution consisting of an allergen is injected into the skin intradermal (intradermal means into the layers of skin and not below the skin). This test is highly sensitive in comparison to the skin prick test. High chances of false positive results prevail in many people who are not allergic to the tested allergen and do not produce any symptoms.

Skin patch test: In this test a pad containing an allergic solution is placed/tagged on the skin for 1-3 days. The skin is observed after 1-3 days. This test easily detects the allergen and is more useful in diagnosis of contact dermatitis.

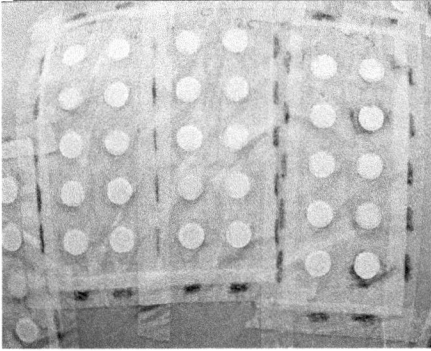

Allergy blood test

Allergy blood tests are done when the skin allergy tests show no response or the patient is not able to undergo skin allergy tests. Allergy blood tests are done for knowing the antibodies produced in the body in response to offensive antigens (allergens here). Antibodies are the substances useful in the defensive mechanism of the body. The blood tests are less sensitive in comparison to allergy skin tests.

Various types of blood tests can be performed to detect the allergen:

- The enzyme-linked immunosorbent assay (ELISA, EIA)

- fluoro-allergosorbent testing (FAST)

- radioallergosorbent testing (RAST)

- Multiple antigen simultaneous testing (MAST)

- An immunoassay capture test (ImmunoCAP, UniCAP, or Pharmacia CAP), etc..

Out of all these tests, the ELISA test is most commonly used where the level of serum IgE is known.

Serum IgE levels are higher in Atopic Dermatitis patients. It controls the immune system's response against allergens. IgE levels are also higher in asthma. IgE are the antibodies (protective substances) that are developed against the antigens (harmful substances). The presence of a higher IgE level in Atopic Dermatitis indicates that the body is fighting against suspected allergens.

Blood tests become useful in detecting the allergens when other skin diseases, rashes or eczema's are severe and widespread throughout the body.

Blood tests are also helpful when the patient is on antihistamines or tricyclic antidepressants. The patient is not able to stop these drugs due to symptomatic relief in itching and the habit-forming side effect of these drugs. These drugs do not allow the allergic reactions to occur even though the patient is sensitive to allergens. Reactions do not appear on the skin as a result of the effect of these drugs.

Blood tests are even done when someone is hypersensitive and shows anaphylactic reactions towards allergy skin tests.

Blood tests are also suggested when the allergy skin tests are positive to many food allergens and the physician wants to decide which food the patient is most allergic to. In these circumstances, the ELISA test becomes very helpful.

2. What preparations need to be done before conducting the tests?

Various medicines can alter the result of the skin allergic tests performed. Hence the patient must convey to the physician all the medicines consumed. The physician should be informed of both nonprescription and prescription medicines. Medicines like tricyclic antidepressants, antihistamines like cetirizine (Zyrtec), fexofenadine (Allegra), and loratadine (Claritin) etc must be discontinued before performing any allergy skin test.

The patient must ask the physician regarding the requirement of the allergy test, types of allergy test, methods of performing the test, risks of the test, side effects (if any) of the test, results of the test and usefulness of the test before proceeding. This will help the patient to get mentally and physically prepared beforehand. It also helps in understanding the utility of the tests and to fill in the medical test information form given to the patient before appearing for the skin allergy tests.

3. How are the skin tests performed?

Before performing the skin prick test and the intradermal test, the site of the test is cleaned with an alcohol swab. The back or arms are usually the preferred sites of performing the test. The allergens or allergen solution is dropped on the skin about 2.5 cm to 5 cm apart. Various allergens can be tested this way at the same time.

In the skin prick test the skin is pricked with a needle where the allergen drop is placed. The pricked needle will allow the allergen to penetrate the skin. The skin prick test can also be performed by using a device which contains 5 to 10 pointed heads that work as needles. The device is dipped into the vessel containing allergen solution and is pierced into the skin of the forearm or back.

In the intradermal test the allergen solution is injected into the skin with the help of a syringe and needle.

The reaction is allowed to take place and the skin is observed after 10 to 15 minutes. If red, raised itchy circles form, the test is positive and the patient is allergic to the allergen.

When the skin prick test is negative but still there is suspicion for the allergen to cause allergic reactions, an intradermal skin test is performed. A skin prick test is usually preferred as an intradermal skin test may cause severe allergic reactions. Both the skin prick test and the intradermal test are completed within 60 minutes.

In the skin patch test the suspected allergen or the allergen solution is placed on patches that are tagged or stuck to the skin. These patches appear like bandages. The preferred site of tagging the patches is the back. Usually 40 minutes are required to tag the patches on the skin. They are worn for 1-3 days. During this period the patient is not allowed to take a bath or do activities that cause excessive perspiration as it may loosen the patches and they may fall off. The patients are strictly not allowed to remove the patches by themselves. The allergists will remove the patches and will observe the allergic reactions (if any).

4. How is the Blood test performed?

The blood test is performed by the expert laboratory technician. The site from which blood is drawn is cleaned with an alcohol swab. The preferred site of withdrawal of blood is cubital fossa (front of elbow). An elastic band is tied around the arm, which will restrict the blood flow towards the arm from the forearm. The veins will get engorged below the band and hence penetrating the needle into the vein becomes easier and quick. The syringe may be used to collect the blood or a tube may be placed near the needle to collect the blood. The band is removed from the arm as soon as the collection of the required amount of blood is completed. A cotton ball dipped in alcohol or spirit is rolled over the prick site after removing the needle. Pressure is applied over the site while rubbing the cotton ball. Then a bandage is tied around the site and the blood sample is sent for antibody tests. If the level of IgE is high, the person is allergic to certain allergens.

5. How does it feel when the allergic tests are done?

A pricking sensation and very mild pain may be felt when the needle penetrates the skin in a skin prick test or intradermal skin test.

If the patient is allergic to an allergen then allergic reactions may occur at the site. Local pain, tenderness, itching, redness and swelling are found. Cool cloths, ice, non-prescription and low potency steroid creams can be applied on the allergen test site to relieve the signs and symptoms of the allergic reactions.

In the case of the skin patch test extreme itching, pain, swelling and redness may occur, on which occasion a physician must be contacted immediately. A severe reaction is found in skin patch tests as the allergens stay on the body for a long time.

In the case of a blood test the patient may feel negligible pricking, stinging or a pinching sensation when the needle is pricked for a blood sample collection. Few patients may feel mild pain when the needle is inserted into the vein. Usually there is no discomfort or pain during or after the blood test is performed.

6. What are the risks associated with skin tests?

Severe anaphylaxis occurs in few patients due to the skin prick test and intradermal test. Anaphylactic reactions have severe symptoms like difficulty in breathing, unconsciousness, swelling of the face and the whole body, severe itching, hypotension (reduced blood pressure) and more. The patient may even die due to anaphylactic reaction. The patient needs to be given emergency aid when any of the symptoms of anaphylaxis are seen. Anaphylaxis is more common in the intradermal test compared to the skin prick test. In the patch test, when patients feel very uncomfortable they must contact the allergist and the treating physician immediately.

In a blood test there are not usually any risks involved. The patient may have minor complaints like bruises and pain at the site of injection. Bruises appear as bluish, reddish or blackish discoloration of the skin. Bruises can be avoided by applying pressure on the punctured site with a cotton swab after withdrawing the needle used for collection of blood.

Phlebitis (inflammation of a vein) may occur in very few patients after puncturing the vein with a needle. Pain and swelling may be seen. It can be treated by applying warm compression and anticoagulant ointments (thrombofob) on the affected area.

Severe, continued bleeding can occur in patients with bleeding disorders like haemophilia (a disease in which the blood does not coagulate and bleeding continues for a while). It may also occur in patients who are on blood thinning medicines like Aspirin, warfarin (Coumadin) etc. Patients must inform the physician if such bleeding disorders prevail or they are on these anticoagulant drugs.

7. What are the results of the allergic tests?

Allergy skin test

The results of the skin prick test and intradermal test are obtained within 1 hour and the result of the skin patch test is obtained after 1-3 days.

In negative allergy skin tests wheals (red raised patch) are not formed.

In positive allergy tests a wheal of 3 mm is formed by the allergen. The bigger the wheal the more allergic the patient is to that particular allergen.

Allergy blood tests

The antibody levels in the allergy blood tests are obtained after 7 days.

In negative allergy blood tests the level of IgE (immunoglobulin E) is not increased. It is same as a normal individual without allergy.

In positive allergy blood tests the levels of IgE for a specific allergen are increased (4 times) in comparison to a normal individual without an allergy.

When are the skin allergy tests not possible?

A skin patch test is not possible or may show abnormal results when the patient sweats extremely and the patch become wet. Skin allergy tests are not possible when the patient has the habit of taking antihistamines or antidepressants.

8. What should be kept in mind before proceeding for the test?

Allergy tests are not required when allergies are mild and do not affect the living of the patient to a great extent. When the allergies are controlled with simple precautions and medicines allergy tests are not required.

However, if allergies affect the daily routine of the patient and they are so severe that they are not controlled with simple medicines then the patient needs to go for allergy tests. Skin allergy tests are simple, easy, and affordable and take around 3-4 hours to get the results. They are more accurate and reliable in comparison to blood allergy tests. The aeroallergens like dust, pollens, animal hairs etc are more precisely detected in skin allergy tests. A skin allergy test cannot conclude food allergies. Food allergy tests are required. Skin allergy tests are not suitable for very young children due to the pricking of the needle.

Blood tests for allergy are expensive in comparison to skin allergy tests. They are less sensitive in comparison to skin tests. They are useful when the skin diseases are widespread throughout the body and the skin allergic reactions in allergic skin tests are difficult to identify. Allergy blood tests are useful also when the person is used to antihistamines and tricyclic antidepressants. Patients can continue the medicines even when the test is performed. They do not initiate any allergic reaction, which is commonly found in the skin allergy test.

Food allergy test

In the food allergy test the person initially has to note down all the food he or she eats daily. Then the food that caused an allergic reaction of any kind must be specifically noted. The identified food is then stopped for 2 weeks. If more than one food caused an allergic reaction then one by one the suspected food must be stopped for 2 weeks. During the restriction period the patient must note down any improvement in the skin or any allergic reaction on the skin. After 2 weeks the food must be reintroduced under the supervision of an expert allergist and physician. If after reintroduction an allergic reaction develops then the patient may be allergic to that specific food. For the confirmation of allergy, a repeat trial of restriction and reintroduction for 2 weeks has to be done. If similar allergic reactions develop which were found previously then the patient is definitely allergic to that specific food. Usually Atopic Dermatitis patients are allergic to soya products, milk products, eggs, shellfish, sour items, wheat flour etc.

Thus these allergy tests help in deciding various allergens, food allergens, sensitive medicines that produce reactions in the patient, toxins etc. It is also helpful in deciding the allergic treatment required for the patient.

Itching is the hallmark symptom of Atopic Dermatitis but it may be found in great severity in other skin diseases like psoriasis, skin infections, contact dermatitis, urticaria, fungal affections and more. Hence if the patient has severe itching, the conclusion cannot be drawn that patient is suffering from Atopic Dermatitis. It is important for the physician to take into consideration other diseases that cause skin irritation and inflammation. Every patient suffers from different and unique symptoms. A single prominent symptom or combination of many symptoms may also be seen. The severity of the disease may also vary from patient to patient. Diagnosis is done on the basis of personal history, family history and unique individual symptoms. For correct information and observation of the patient, the physician may need to see the patient many times so that no small information is missed. A family doctor or pediatrician of a child may seek the opinion of an expert dermatologist or allergist for correct diagnosis and treatment.

Chapter 7: Treating Atopic Dermatitis Conventionally

Treatment of Atopic Dermatitis can be done by joint efforts between the treating doctor, the patient and family members of the patient. Before starting the treatment, the physician usually counsels the patient to remain calm during the treatment. Aggression, irritability and unnecessary stress must be avoided, as it becomes a hindrance in the way of a cure. Night watching must not be done and healthy, fresh food must be consumed. The treating physician counsels the patient about his/her condition and the appearance of the skin. The signs and symptoms will be relieved, but the patient needs to have patience for relief.

The treating physician will commence the treatment by forming a treatment plan. It is planned on the basis of the patient's age, presenting signs and symptoms, personal history, family history, pattern of onset of symptoms, age at which symptoms began, aggravating and ameliorating factors, other diseases like diabetes, hypertension, cardiac diseases, psychological disease, etc., and the present and general health of the patient. The treatment plan is conveyed to the patient and family members. The patient and family members must religiously follow the treatment plan. The success of the treatment plan greatly depends on how carefully the patient and the family members follow the instructions and act accordingly.

In the beginning, the majority of patients of Atopic Dermatitis are not given intensive care. Dressings can be done for the lesions. Wet bandages are tied on the affected site for 30 minutes. This prevents external irritants coming into contact with the lesions and deteriorating them.

Patients are managed on a conservative basis and are advised to take proper skin care. They are taught how to take good care of their skin and are advised to avoid harmful sunrays, severely polluted atmospheres, extremely cold or hot weather, harsh cosmetics, etc. The patient is also advised to avoid night watching, alcohol drinking, cigarette smoking, pungent food, stale food and severe exercise. Patients are easily managed at home. A lot of improvement is seen by applying non-fragrant, chemical free, natural lubricants on the face, hands and all over the body after bathing. These lubricants prevent moisture loss and dryness. Moisturizers can be applied during the day and night after bathing, when the body is slightly wet. This helps to lock natural moisture into the skin. Itching is greatly relieved when the skin's moisture is retained. Dry skin has an itchy tendency. Coal tar applications can be helpful in relieving itching, but they should not be applied on irritated skin. If no benefit is found after an application for itching, it should be discontinued. It works best after the lesions have been suppressed with other external applications and medications.

Usually with the help of conservative treatment, the lesions heal within three weeks.

The treatment of Atopic Dermatitis is planned in such a way that the following main goals are achieved:

1) To heal the damaged skin;

2) To revive and renew the skin and make it healthy;

3) To maintain the health of the skin;

4) To prevent the flaring and relapse of the disease;

5) To provide relief and treatment when the signs and symptoms recur.

Skin care is given great emphasis in treatment. Skin care can be achieved by forming good habits in the care of the skin. It should become a daily routine that needs to be followed religiously. Those factors that exacerbate the disease and those stimulants which trigger the "itch- scratch" cycle must be first identified and then avoided as much as possible. Those circumstances and surroundings that activate the immune system of the skin must be strictly avoided.

The hyperactive immune system of the patient responds severely to the least stimuli and reacts aggressively, which leads to hypersensitive reactions like excessive, uncontrolled itching, scratching, swelling and redness. Sometimes more than one treatment plan is also developed in advanced cases, relapsing cases and unresponsive cases of the disease. Every minute change in appearance, inflammation, signs and symptoms must be noted by the patient or the relatives. No minute change should be left unnoticed after commencing treatment. It should be carefully observed whether the color of the lesion has changed, inflammation has reduced or increased, itching is relieved or has increased, etc.

All these changes regarding the skin can help the physician in determining the correct condition of the skin, severity of the disease, response to treatment, necessary changes in the treatment if required, underlying disease of the body other than Atopic Dermatitis, differential diagnosis of the other diseases in the body that may be aggravating or maintaining the Atopic Dermatitis, planning of the subsequent treatment for both Atopic Dermatitis and underlying disease, prognosis of the disease, etc. Hence for the physician's assistance and speedy improvement, none of the minute changes in the skin should be ignored. They should be noted so that they are not forgotten.

Skin care must be kept simple and the basic regimen should be followed. Unnecessary fuss and complication should be avoided. Combining too many methods for skin care could ultimately harm the skin instead of improving it. The key to the best skin care is to keep it simple and easy. Simple and easy methods can be practiced for long periods of time and the patient does not become tired of using them. Complicated, combined methods used for short periods do not show any improvement, whereas simple methods practiced for long periods show excellent results. Simple regimens like the use of mild soap and one moisturizer prescribed by the physician should be followed.

Use of multiple soaps, lotions, moisturizers, perfumes, deodorants, cosmetics and a mixture of various products harm the skin instead of benefitting it. They arouse new skin problems and the skin becomes more sensitive to external stimuli. A combination of various products does not allow any product to work properly with full effect. Combined products may even interact with each other and cause serious allergic reactions and harm the skin. Severe redness, itching, swelling, pigmentation on the skin and other side effects may arise due to a combination of various external applications. The hypersensitive skin of the Atopic Dermatitis patient immediately shows profound side effects, which take a long time to recover. Circumstances may arise where the treating physician will have to treat the side effects of the various products instead of the lesions of Atopic Dermatitis.

It may happen that when one prescribed product starts giving a good result, the patient may discontinue it due to many reasons and start using another product. Hence the full benefit of the prescribed product is not obtained. This may dishearten the patient and he/she starts feeling that it is not improving. Results-oriented products may end up in showing no result just because the patient either discontinues it abruptly or starts applying a mixture of products. Enough time should be given to any one product to show visible results. It must be kept in mind that the prescribed applications are medicinal products, and not magic that will show improvement overnight. Hence it is advisable for the patient to follow one product prescribed by the physician for a reasonable period of time without combining it with other applications. Efforts are made on the part of the physician to heal the skin, make it healthy and to keep it healthy for a longer period of time.

Healthy skin is not easily susceptible to harmful pathogens,

polluted surroundings, allergic substances and all other irritating
and annoying environmental stimuli. Healthy skin resists the
notorious stimulus and does not allow it to cause harmful effects.
More damage to the hypersensitive skin of the Atopic Dermatitis
patient is prevented by healthy, healing skin.

Patients are encouraged when visible improvements are seen on
the skin and the quality of life is greatly improved. The
confidence levels of patients are greatly increased when lesions
start healing and healthy skin replaces the ugly looking lesions of
Atopic Dermatitis. For quick healing and healthy skin, the daily
skin care routine developed by the physician needs to be
followed. A bath should be taken daily. Many Atopic Dermatitis
patients avoid daily bathing. This will allow the accumulation of
dirt, dust, sand, perspiration, etc., on the body, which will
aggravate severe itching, scratching and inflammation.
Maintaining cleanliness is of the utmost importance in the
treatment of Atopic Dermatitis.

1. Initial regimen

The initial regimen consists of bathing and moisturizing.

a. Bathing

Baths should be taken in a proper way. Very hot water should not
be used in bathing. Hot water causes dryness of the skin and it
may prove irritating for many people. The natural moisture and
oil of the skin is drained away due to excessive hot water. Rashes
may appear on the skin, and many people develop urticaria (red or
white hives) on the body after a hot bath. In bitter winters, too,
use of excessive hot water in bathing should be avoided.
Similarly, very cold water also should not be used. Very cold
water also causes dryness of the skin. It may cause
vasoconstriction (constriction of small blood vessels supplying
blood, oxygen and nutrition to the skin) of capillaries, and hence
the natural healing of the lesions does not occur. Reduced blood
supply to the skin does not allow phagocytes (white blood cells
involved in the defense mechanism of the body) to accumulate

around lesions and induce healing activity. The oxygen supply may be reduced in the skin, causing health issues.

Hence instead of very hot or cold water, lukewarm water is preferable. In circumstances when the patient is outdoors, travelling, ill, bedridden, hospitalized or due to any other reason, bathing is not possible, then sponging with lukewarm water must be done. One tablespoon or capful of chlorine bleach can be added to lukewarm water. Chlorine bleach helps in the cleaning of the body. It removes dust, debris and sweat thoroughly. It also has a disinfectant property and hence it does not allow harmful microorganisms to grow in the water or on the skin. Secondary infection with pathogens such as bacteria, virus, fungi, spores, etc. can be prevented with the use of chlorine bleach. It is cheap and readily available in all grocery and medicinal shops.

However, the treating physician should always be consulted before its use. Prolonged bathing is to be avoided. Baths taken for a long time cause prolonged dampness on the skin. Normal bathing time for Atopic Dermatitis patient ranges from 10-20 minutes. Bathing should be done gently and not vigorously. Gentle rubbing of the skin is to be done with the hands. A piece of cloth or sponge must not be used for bathing, as it is rough for the sensitive skin. Generally a mild, gentle bar soap, soap-free body wash or natural cleansers are advised. Harsh soaps should be totally avoided as they cause severe drying of the skin. After bathing with harsh soaps, the patient feels as if the skin is stretched, which leads to itching and scratching.

Mild, gentle scrubs can be used while bathing. An oatmeal bath is considered very useful and refreshing for the patient. Scrubs like oatmeal, walnut skin extracts, cinnamon powder, millet flour, lentil flour, etc., are naturally available and they should be used. They can be easily prepared at home and are free from any artificial chemicals. They can be rubbed on the skin in a circular manner. This will remove dead skin cells and will increase skin circulation. Toxins and allergens will be removed and the skin is revived.

Bathing in seawater should be avoided as far as possible because seawater is harsh, salty and full of minerals that may prove to be irritable for the patient's hypersensitive skin. Even bathing in a swimming pool is also not advisable as it contains very high levels of chlorine, which aggravate itching. Atopic Dermatitis is not contagious and it does not spread to other people by bathing in a swimming pool. But if secondary infection is present with microorganisms, it becomes contagious and spreads to other people bathing in the same swimming pool.

b. Moisturizing

Once bathing is complete, an effective emollient cream should be applied all over the body. It should be immediately applied while the skin is slightly wet. Towel drying of the skin is to be avoided as the natural moisture of the water is lost by vigorous towel drying. A good quality emollient or cream that has a thick, stiff consistency should be used. Thick emollients do not move out or drop from the jar when opened and inverted. They lock in the natural moisture of the skin and restore natural oils that are lost during bathing. They also inhibit evaporation of water from the skin when the patient moves outdoors in the sun and open air. Creams and emollients are very helpful for the quick healing of skin lesions. They prevent dryness of the skin, which is the key to quick healing. They establish a protective barrier between environmental stimuli and the hypersensitive skin.

A thick layer of creams and emollients does not allow harmful pathogens and irritants to easily penetrate the skin, which prevents damage to it. Moreover, the use of emollients makes the patients feel good throughout the day as they find the skin soft, supple and itch free. Natural, chemical-free body butters can also be used. Emollients prepared from tar are used in healing of very dry, lichenified areas of the body. Petroleum jelly preparations can be freely applied all over the body. Emollients enriched with vitamin E and other essential oils can also be used. Vitamin E and other essential oils enhance the healing power of emollients.

Whichever cream or emollient is chosen, it must not possess any fragrance or artificial, harsh chemicals. Artificial, fragrant substances may induce allergic reactions and worsen the symptoms of the patient. The patient is always tempted to use them, but they should be avoided for long-term benefit. Emollients used must be waterproof. They should not drain away while washing your hands, legs or face. Only emollients should be used that are well proven and are prescribed by the physician. The use of lotions is not recommended as they have high water or alcohol content. Alcohol and water quickly evaporate upon coming into contact with atmospheric air and sunlight. They also have liquid consistency, which does not form a thick layer on the skin. They are usually not waterproof, and hence a protective barrier is not formed.

For healthy skin, patients must be cautious and alert all the time about the skin condition. Any minute change in the skin should be noticed and conveyed to the treating physician. For protecting and restoring healthy skin, infections are to be avoided. However, it is practically not possible to avoid all infections and allergens that are present in the surrounding environment. For preventing infections the patient must avoid going into highly contaminated zones, severely polluted areas and crowded places. Even after enough precautions, if infection sets in on any part of the body, it should not be ignored.

Patients should immediately seek the physician's advice on noting the development of infection on the body. Early signs and symptoms of the infection must be identified by the patient and the relatives. Small blisters or papules may appear on the arms, legs, trunk, back or face. They are yellowish to greenish in appearance and sometimes may be bright red or inflamed. They may ooze fluid, serum or pus. The discharge may be foul smelling. Crusty, scaly areas may form around the infected site. The pus becomes irritable for the patients and they scratch the infected site severely and repeatedly. Bleeding may occur and thus healing is prevented. The progress of the infection can be aborted and the harmful effects of the infection can be minimized if the infections are identified early.

The patient and the relatives must learn how to identify the initial signs and symptoms of secondary infection. They must be able to differentiate the signs and symptoms of Atopic Dermatitis and secondary infection with pathogens. They must acquire this knowledge from the treating physician so that secondary infection does not worsen and prevent healing. The treatment is started as soon as possible and is continued until the complete disappearance of the secondary infection. If required, aggressive therapy is given by the physician for the secondary infection so that it does not flare up.

c. Wet wraps and cooling pads

After applying emollients and topical steroids on the lesions, cooling pads and wet bandages are wrapped on the affected site. It is preferable to use elastic bandages, as they are more convenient to the patient. Wet bandages and cooling pads become very help-ful when the eczema is severely hot, itchy and red. The wet ban-dages and cooling pads relieve burning, itching and fasten the process of healing. They moisturize the skin and prevent dryness. It also prevents scratching of the skin as the lesions are covered with a bandage. They can be applied several times a day and can be continued according to the requirements of the patient. The bandage needs to be changed when they dry out.

Moreover, the signs and symptoms of any other disease in the body should be given importance. No disease involving any system of the body should be ignored. Underlying diabetes mellitus, hypertension, autoimmune disease or infection in vital organs may flare up Atopic Dermatitis and prevent its cure. Hence all the minute details must be conveyed to the treating physician.

2. When to Visit the Doctor?

The doctor should be consulted immediately when the itching becomes severe and it interferes with the routine activity of the patient. This is when the patient becomes uncomfortable at home, school and work and is not able to sleep at night. The lesions cover up the whole body and oozing becomes profound, along with bleeding. Secondary infection sets in and high-grade fever occurs. In these circumstances the patient should visit the doctor.

Who can be Contacted for the Treatment of Atopic Dermatitis?

The patient can contact any of the following:

1) A family doctor

2) A physician

3) A pediatrician

4) A dermatologist

5) An allergist

6) Alternative treatment therapist

These treating people can interconnect with each other and commence the treatment. The family doctor can refer the patient to an expert dermatologist or allergist.

What are the Points One Should Bear in Mind Before Visiting the Physician and During Subsequent Therapy?

Honesty must be the first thing the patient should keep in mind when visiting the physician. No wrong information about the disease should be conveyed to the physician. True information provided by the patient is of utmost importance as the physician prepares the treatment plan according to the signs and symptoms narrated by the patient. The patient should convey the exact information about the disease. Information must neither be exaggerated nor be undervalued by the patient. For example, if the patient has severe itching at night he/she should not undervalue this symptom and must convey it to the physician, as it is a prominent symptom of Atopic Dermatitis. The patient may consider complaints as routine, but they may be of great value for diagnosis, treatment and prognosis of the disease.

Another example is if the patient is sensitive to the sun and it produces tanning and redness on the skin when staying out for along time in the sun, then the patient should convey this information to the physician. However, it should not be conveyed in an exaggerated manner that on least exposure to sun severe itching, redness, swelling, burning, etc., develops. This exaggerated information provided by the patient will confuse the physician who may decide to provide phototherapy to the patient even though he or she may not require it or will not be greatly benefited by it. No signs and symptoms should be missed by the patient. For that, patients must write down on a piece of paper complaints they are suffering from and should carry it while visiting the physician. In this way, no signs or symptoms will be missed that are required for diagnosis, treatment and prognosis of the disease.

Complete information about the disease is to be narrated to the physician.

- How it started?

- What were the initial symptoms?

- On which part did the first signs and symptoms appear?

- At which age did the first lesion develop?

- Were there any periods of flare or remission?

- Did the disease subside after a few months of age?

- How did it reappear?

- On reappearance were the symptoms very severe or mild?

- Was any treatment taken previously?

- Do any other family members suffer from the disease?

- Do the first relatives have any other major skin disease?

- Is there any other major disease presently in the body?

- Has any major disease occurred in the past?

- Was any hospitalization done previously?

- Is there any allergy present in the body?

- Is there any drug that causes allergic reactions?

- Is any external application being applied or not?

- Has any secondary infection appeared at any time?

- What was the treatment taken for secondary infections?

- Are there any periods of depression?

- Is there any particular time when the signs and symptoms are aggravated by themselves and get relieved spontaneously?

- In which season are the majority of symptoms relieved or aggravated?

- Is there only one prominent symptom or group of symptoms?

- What is the lifestyle and daily routine?

- Is there any maintaining cause present in the daily routine?

- Is there any known triggering factor?

- Is there any food allergy?

- Was any alternative therapy previously taken or is currently ongoing?

- How is the residing place?

- How often is cleaning done?

- Are there any pets in the house?

- What is the occupation?

All this information must be answered by the patient himself or herself if they are an adult and must be conveyed correctly to the physician.

In the case of infants and children, all this information must be conveyed by the mother or the person taking care of the child. The mother should closely observe the child daily so that even a slight change is not overlooked and is conveyed to the physician. The mother should be very cautious of secondary infection, which may develop at any time on lesions of Atopic Dermatitis. She should immediately contact the physician about it. If the child is older and is able to narrate complaints, then he/she should be encouraged to do so.

Patients should always bring a list of queries and concerns they have about the disease when they visit the physician. It may happen that the patient forgets to ask important questions during the visit if the list is not made in advance. Commonly asked questions include the following:

- Is Atopic Dermatitis is a serious disease?

- Is the present condition curable?

- What is the duration in which the symptoms will be relieved?

- Will it take very long for relief or will it be relieved within a short period?

- Would the relief be temporary or permanent?

- Will the disease spread to other family members in the house?

- Is isolation required?

- What kind of treatment is to be given?

- Is the treatment a repetition of previously taken treatment?

- Are there any agents in the treatment that may have side effects?

- Will the side effects be temporary or have long lasting effects?

- Is there any way to avoid the side effects?

- What are the precautions that are needed when the treatment is going on?

- Is there any requirement for taking leave from work?

- What kind of diet is to be taken during the therapy?

- Are there any dietary restrictions to be kept?

- What kind of soaps and cosmetics can be used?

- Are cosmetics required to be avoided completely?

- Is there any requirement for hospitalization?

- Can any alternative therapy be used along with the main line of treatment?

- How effective can alternative therapy be?

- What are the chances of recurrence?

- What precautions can be taken to prevent recurrence?

- Can breastfeeding be given to a baby when the lesions are around the nipples?

Likewise, many other questions can be asked by adult patients to the physician so that they become well aware about the condition and the precautions to be kept while the treatment is going on.

3. Pharmacotherapy

a. Coal tar preparations

Coal tar preparations can be generously applied on the body and the affected areas as an initial treatment. They relieve inflammation and itching of the skin. Coal tar applications should be cautiously used as they may irritate the skin. They can be used alone or mixed with topical corticosteroids for application. The tar preparations are freely available as over the counter products. Some of the formulations of coal tar contain alcohol in it, which can cause irritation on the skin. The alcohol level is high in the gel form of coal tar preparations, hence they should be avoided. Coal tar shampoos, body washes and creams are safer in comparison to gel form and they do not irritate the skin. Coal tar preparations have a peculiar odor and cause stains on the skin and clothes, hence many people do not choose to use coal tar preparations.

b. Corticosteroid ointments and creams:

The cases of Atopic Dermatitis are usually managed with corticosteroid creams and ointments. They are available as over the counter products as well prescription products. Over the counter products are usually tried and applied by the patient before they consult the physician. Self- medication in the form of application of over the counter corticosteroids is very common. The majority of patients are only temporarily relieved by their use and the symptoms relapse. Over the counter products do not have high-strength of steroids in them. Low strength is found and repeated application of these products may develop resistance in the patient.

Hence the physician usually prescribes a higher strength corticosteroid cream or ointment for topical application (external application on the skin) when the patient comes for treatment. In many patients, allergic reactions may be seen on the application site of corticosteroid creams or ointments. Aggravation instead of relief of the skin symptoms may occur. This happens as the base used in the preparation of corticosteroid creams and ointments may be of low quality or it may be an allergen or irritant for that particular patient. For these patients, corticosteroid ointments that are well proven, branded and with a different base should be used.

Corticosteroid ointments and creams are freely applied by the patient on a regular basis because it greatly relieves symptoms. After the first few applications only, patients start feeling relief in itching, scratching, redness, swelling etc. The lesions quickly start disappearing but they may easily reappear. Patients usually overuse the topical corticosteroids.

Hence, side effects develop after long-term use. Common side effects of topical corticosteroids include: 1) thinning of the skin, 2) secondary infections with microorganisms, 3) suppression of the disease, 4) spread of disease to deeper vital organs, 5) suppression of normal growth in children, 6) stretch marks on the skin, 7) atrophy of blood vessels of skin, etc. After abuse of topical steroids, the episodes of flare-ups are more severe and difficult to treat.

c. Immunomodulators

Calcineurin inhibitors like tacrolimus (Protopic) and pimecrolimus (Elidel) ointments are used for treatment next. They are new topical immunomodulators. Immunomodulators work by altering the immune system of the patient. Atopic Dermatitis patients have a hyperactive immune system, which reacts aggressively to even less powerful stimuli. The powerful topical medicated ointments work by mildly modulating and suppressing the immune system of the Atopic Dermatitis patient. When tacrolimus and pimecrolimus are applied on intact skin in limited and reasonable amounts, they do not cause any harm. They do not cause any major alteration in the immune system of the body. They are not very useful in treating severe disease or severely flared up periods in adults. They work very well on mild lesions, especially on the faces of children.

These immunomodulators are commonly used in oral form in patients undergoing kidney and liver transplantation. These drugs help the body to accept the new transplanted kidney or liver. They suppress the immune system and do not allow the body to give a foreign body reaction when the organs are received. Hence the transplant of the kidney or liver is not rejected by the body and treatment becomes successful.

These immunomodulator ointments do not cause thinning of the skin, atrophy of blood vessels or skin, stretch marks or other harm to the skin in comparison to topical steroids. The Food and Drug Administration (FDA) of America has issued a warning that these immunomodulators should be avoided, or if unavoidable, they should be used very cautiously. They may harm the body by extensively suppressing the immune system. It may happen that the natural immune response that is required for fighting against harmful stimulus is also suppressed. Hence a variety of diseases involving various systems of the body may occur. Some reports suggest that these drugs may cause skin cancers and cancer in other parts of the body. Even though the warning is issued by the FDA, dermatologists and other physicians prescribe these drugs for children and adults. They prescribe the drugs in safe dosages, taking into consideration the severity of the disease and the general health of the patient.

The physician generally discusses all the pros and cons of the treatment with the patient before commencing the treatment, so that the patient is aware of any possible side effects and may immediately contact the physician for treatment.

d. Barrier repair devices

Atopiclair and MimyX creams are combined with topical steroids and emollients and are applied all over the body. These creams have been recently introduced for treatment. They are used both in adults and children. They make a protective shield on the skin. They enhance the barrier function of the skin and protect the skin against harmful pathogens and allergic stimulants. The protective shield does not allow evaporation of moisture from the skin so natural moisture is retained in the skin. Dryness of the skin is greatly relieved with the use of these drugs. The skin of the Atopic Dermatitis patient is usually broken due to severe scratching and rubbing. It gets repaired with the use of these topical creams.

e. Antibiotics

Symptomatic treatment is given for various signs and symptoms of the disease. Antibiotics are used when secondary bacterial infections of Streptococcus, Staphylococcus, S. Aureus, etc., occur. They are used in oral and topical form. Topical antibacterial ointments are applied directly on the lesions of the skin. Topical antibacterial ointments give satisfactory results if the lesions are small and not grossly affected with bacteria. If lesions are deeply affected, extensive pus discharge is found, severe pain is felt, crusty lesions are developed and/or inflammation is greatly increased, then oral antibiotics are to be given. Oral antibiotics in the form of tablets and capsules are more effective in comparison to topical antibiotics in resolving the symptoms.

Intravenous and intramuscular antibiotics are given in the form of injections and drips. They are used when extensive, heavy bacterial infection is found. Fever, vomiting, headache, pain, malaise, general debility, etc., occurs. A superficial bacterial infection penetrates the skin deeply and causes a systemic infection, which affects the vital organs of the body. The penicillin group of drugs: macrolids like erythromycin, azithromycin; cephalosporins like cephalexin, etc., are the commonly used antibiotics for secondary bacterial infections.

f. Antiviral

In raw, open and broken skin, a secondary viral infection may also occur. Viral infections like herpes simplex, herpes zoster, etc. set in. Herpes infections usually occur around the lips, genitals and the back. Small, fluid filled blisters and papules occur. Severe burning and pain is the hallmark of a herpes infection. Herpes has a rapid course and flares up overnight. A secondary infection of herpes should be immediately treated, as it is very annoying for the patient. Oral and topical antiviral medication is administered. Acyclovir ointment and tablets are commonly used for herpes infections.

g. Antifungal

Secondary fungal infections may also occur in broken, open skin. Dry or wet fungal infections may set in with severe itching. The ozole group of drugs like ketacanazole, flucanazole; terbinafine, etc., are used for fungal infections. They are used both in oral and topical form.

h. Antihistaminic drugs

Night aggravation of itching, scratching and rubbing is usually found in all the patients of the Atopic Dermatitis. Antihistaminic drugs are given to relieve itching. Antihistaminic drugs like phenaramine maleate, chlorphenarimine maleate, citrizine, levocitrizine, etc., are commonly used. Antihistamines induce drowsiness in the patient and help the patient to have a sound sleep at night, which greatly benefits the patients as they have a sense of wellbeing after good sleep. Patients feel energetic and they may be able to concentrate more at work the next morning.

Sound sleep helps in building up the natural immunity of the person, which may further benefit the patient. Itching and scratching is also greatly relieved due to antihistamines. Due to reduced scratching at nighttime the skin becomes less raw and thus inflammation is reduced. Antihistamines should be taken at nighttime before going to bed. During the daytime they should be avoided as they cause drowsiness.

The patient may feel sleepy throughout the day if taken in the morning. It is not necessary that antihistamines may benefit all patients, so it should be continued only if relief is found.

i. Leukotriene inhibitors

The leukotriene inhibitors are commonly used for treatment of asthma. They are also effective in allergic disorders like wheezing and sneezing. Asthma and Atopic Dermatitis have allergic predisposition hence drugs used for asthma may be also used for Atopic Dermatitis. Therefore leukotrienes inhibitors may be considered for use in Atopic Dermatitis. Commonly used leukotriene inhibitors include zileuton, zafirlukast, montelukast etc. Few reports have shown some improvement in the skin condition of the patient. Zafirlukast shows good results but should not be given to children under 12 years of age. Montelukast must be avoided in very young children (less than 6 years).

j. Antineoplastic drugs

Antineoplastic drugs may be of some benefit to a Atopic Dermatitis patient. In a study, 24 patients suffering from Atopic Dermatitis were given human interferon gamma (antineoplastic drug) for trial. These patients were given the drug for 2 years and all the patients showed improvement. No significant side effects were observed. The anti neoplastic drugs like Cyclosporine, methotrexate, azathioprine, mycophenolate, mofetil etc may be used in advanced cases. However, intense studies and experiments are lacking for the use of antineoplastic drugs. Placebo studies are not done. In a few other studies conducted no improvement was also noted.

Still the role of atnineoplastic drugs in the treatments is an area where further research and more evidence based practice is needed.

k. Anesthetic creams

Anaesthetic creams may be used to relieve itching, burning and pain of the lesions. Anaesthetic creams like mixture of 5% lidocaine and 5% prilocaine are applied on the affected site. When these anaesthetics are applied for 5-15 min on dry eczema, blanching (the skin appears white) occurs and pain and itching is relieved. However, if the anaesthetics are applied for 30-60 min on eczema then the skin becomes very red or red spots may be seen. This occurs due to rapid absorption of anaesthetics in the skin. Hence it is preferable to apply it for a shorter time.

l. Antiseptic solutions

Antiseptic solutions can be applied on eczemas that are infected with microorganisms (bacteria). Antiseptic solutions must not be very concentrated. Concentrated solutions can irritate the skin. Along with antiseptic solutions, emollients and moisturizers must be applied. Common examples of antiseptic solutions are cetrimide, chlorhexidine, chloroxylenol, dibromopropamidine, polynoxylin, povidone iodine and triclosan. They are mixed with bath water. They prevent bacterial growth and further deterioration of lesions.

½ cup of 6% sodium hypochlorite solution (bleach) is added to water and this water can be used for bathing. Affected skin can be soaked for 10 minutes in the bleach water.

Weak potassium permanganate (Condy's crystals) that is not very concentrated can be added in bathing water. It should be added less in quantity, just enough to make the water light pink in color.

4. Phototherapy

Phototherapy can also be used for treatment of Atopic Dermatitis. The patient is exposed to ultraviolet light for a prescribed and reasonable amount of time. Phototherapy may not suit everyone. Phototherapy is not suitable for the patients who are allergic to sunrays. Patients whose redness, swelling, itching and burning increases when exposed to sunrays should not take phototherapy. If patients have a history of flared eczema due to sun exposure, sun induced skin problems, sunstroke on least exposure to the sun then they should not be given phototherapy. It is employed to children over 12 years and adults. It is not given to infants and younger children.

Phototherapy is usually never employed alone. It is always given in combination with regular treatment of Atopic Dermatitis. Along with phototherapy, conservative treatment of Atopic Dermatitis consisting of mild soap, moisturizing emollients, creams, corticosteroid creams, oral corticosteroids (if required), etc., must be employed. Maintaining and triggering causes are also required to be managed while employing phototherapy. If they persist, phototherapy will not show any good relief. Along with Atopic Dermatitis, phototherapy is also used to treat many other skin conditions like seborrheic dermatitis, psoriasis and other types of eczema. Phototherapy is given when the lesions of Atopic Dermatitis are not very severe. It does not show effective results when the lesions are widespread and require extensive therapy. It works very well in the case of mild to moderate Atopic Dermatitis.

Phototherapy consists of two major types. One type is ultraviolet light therapy and the other is ultraviolet A therapy along with psoralen (a type of medicine). Ultraviolet A therapy with psoralen is also known as chemophototherapy or PUVA therapy.

In ultraviolet light therapy, ultraviolet A or ultraviolet B rays are employed on the skin of the affected person. The rays may be employed all over the body or only on lesions of Atopic Dermatitis. Light waves may contain only ultraviolet A or only ultraviolet B rays. A combination of both can also be used. The light waves can be given directly on the body or after applying coal tar generously all over the body. Applying coal tar may reduce the possible redness, swelling, and rashes that develop after the exposure to light waves. Coal tar soothes the hypersensitive skin of the Atopic Dermatitis patient. Light therapy is always given under the supervision of a dermatologist. It should not be taken at home. While giving UVA and UVB waves, special care of the eyes is taken. Precaution is taken that harmful UVA or UVB waves are not exposed directly to the eyes. Patients are made to wear goggles while taking light therapy.

UVB light therapy further consists of two subdivisions: 1) Broadband UVB therapy and 2) Narrowband UVB therapy. Broadband UVB therapy is given three to five times a week whereas narrowband UVB therapy is given two to three times a week. Broadband therapy is an older form of therapy. It has shown high efficacy in reducing lesions of Atopic Dermatitis for many decades. The patient requires taking the therapy three to five times in a week, which may be difficult for many patients to manage as they have to spare time and travel for taking the treatment. It may even produce severe burning. In some cases skin cancer has been reported to occur after giving broadband UVB therapy. Broadband therapy usually reaches all the parts of the body except deeper areas like the scalp and folds of the inguinal region (pubic folds), elbows, back of knees, etc.

In narrowband UVB therapy, narrow bands of UVB rays are emitted on the skin of the patient. It is a newer therapy in comparison to broadband therapy and it is more effective in healing the lesions. Faster results are found and patients usually find it more convenient as it is required to be taken only two to three times a week. It does not produce severe burning, which is usually found when broadband therapy is employed. The risk of developing skin cancer is also reduced with narrow band UVB rays.

In some cases resistance to ultraviolet light therapy is found. No positive outcome is found even in minor lesions if the patient is resistant to light therapy. In severely resistant cases, instead of phototherapy alone, a newer method known as photochemotherapy or PUVA is employed. Here UVA rays are exposed on the skin of the patient after application of psoralen on the skin.

Psoralen is a medicine that enhances the effect of light therapy and makes the skin more sensitive to UVA rays. Psoralen is applied all over the body and if required it is given in the form of an oral medicine before commencing the treatment. A psoralen bath is usually given. Photochemotherapy with PUVA is given for a long period of time, usually for six months. Several sittings are required to be given. Precaution must be taken to protect the eyes when the therapy is employed. The patient is made to wear goggles (which provide protection against UVA light waves) during the therapy as well as after the therapy for the whole day. Psoralen remains in the eyes for one day and it increases the sensitivity towards UVA rays.

The common side effects of PUVA therapy include nausea, headache throughout the day of therapy, prostration, severe burning and itching skin and irregular blackish, reddish pigmentation all over the body.

Photochemotherapy is employed only for those patients who are sensitive to psoralen and phototherapy. If resistance is found against psoralen, PUVA therapy will have no effect. Many studies have suggested that the patients that are resistant to PUVA can be treated by adding a topical steroid to PUVA therapy. Topical steroids may be applied all over the body before giving PUVA therapy. Positive results are obtained in reducing the lesions.

Phototherapy works by altering the immune system. The hyperactive immune response of the Atopic Dermatitis patient is greatly reduced by applying phototherapy in a particular dose and for a specific period of time. The inflammatory reaction of the lesion is reduced when light waves are employed and this results in redness, swelling, pain and itching. Phototherapy plays a very good role in preventing secondary bacterial infections in an Atopic Dermatitis patient. UVA and UVB rays are considered to be the best sterilizers in the world, as they do not allow the growth of microorganisms on the skin. Microorganisms cannot withstand against UVA and UVB rays. Phototherapy also helps in reducing the use of topical steroids in relieving the lesions of Atopic Dermatitis. In some cases only phototherapy is sufficient and there is no need to use topical steroids.

In unavoidable circumstances where topical steroids are a must, at that time conjoint phototherapy reduces the strength of the topical steroids. However, the effect of phototherapy is different for every patient. Some may have no benefit at all, some may have improvement in signs and symptoms, and some may be completely cured within three weeks of therapy. Hence, varied results are found.

Before applying phototherapy, several points are to be looked for, and then only the therapy is applied. The patients' general health, personal history of sun allergy, family history of sun allergy, medical history of harmful effects of sun, like stroke, skin cancer, etc., history of previous treatment taken, present condition of the skin, history of previously taken phototherapy with its effect, age of the patient are noted. All these points help the dermatologist to know whether the person is the right candidate for phototherapy or not, whether he/she would be able to withstand the therapy with minimal side effects or whether his/her present condition will flare up after the use of the therapy. After analyzing all these points and considering the risks, side effects and benefits of the treatment, if the physician feels that phototherapy may be useful in treating the symptoms of Atopic Dermatitis, he/she will use the minimum amount of rays necessary and will monitor the skin carefully.

Phototherapy is carried out only under the guidance and strict supervision of a dermatologist who is trained in employing the therapy. If the therapy is not employed in the correct dosage, correct area, and correct time and for the correct duration, then it may cause serious side effects like premature ageing of skin, burning, severe rashes, flare of the Atopic Dermatitis lesions and skin cancer.

In circumstances where no response is found from any other method employed, and when the condition of the patient is such that he or she needs to be relieved quickly from the symptoms, then systemic corticosteroids are given. In certain cases the flare-up phase of the disease is so severe that the patient is under severe suffering and the physician is compelled to use systemic corticosteroids. Systemic corticosteroids can be given orally, intramuscularly (given in muscles) or intravenously (given in a blood vein) via tablets, injections or pints (bottle). Systemic steroids are used only in refractory cases and stubborn cases that show the least or no improvement after all other possible therapies are tried. Systemic therapy is never employed in the beginning of treatment. They are added at a very late stage and given only if required. Systemic steroids are avoided in children as much as possible. However, if it is unavoidable, then they are given in minimal dose according to the age, height, weight and the general condition of the child. They are given for a very short period of time and discontinued as soon as improvement is noticed.

Precautions should also be taken when discontinuing systemic steroids. They cannot be abruptly stopped. They are started gradually in increasing doses and are stopped gradually in tapering doses. If systemic corticosteroids are abruptly stopped, they may give rise to severe side effects and flaring of the disease. Commonly prescribed corticosteroids in Atopic Dermatitis are prednisone, betamethasone, etc.

The commonly found side effects of systemic corticosteroids include: 1) severe damage to skin, 2) rough, thin, loose, elastic skin, 3) weak bones, 4) brittle bones, 5) raised blood pressure, 6) diabetes mellitus, 7) respiratory infections, 8) eye infections, 9) development of cataract, 10) increased body weight, 11) hair loss,

12) overgrowth in children, 13) obesity in children to name but a few. Systemic corticosteroids employed via tablets have fewer side effects than those employed via injections or pints. The majority of patients improve dramatically after using systemic corticosteroids. Redness, swelling, itching and scratching is typically completely relieved.

There are a few patients in whom even systemic corticosteroids do not show any improvement and topical corticosteroids, systemic corticosteroids, emollients, and phototherapy have very little effect. In these patients, immunosuppressive drugs are employed. Immunosuppressive drugs are employed in adults only. They are never given to children. The common examples of immunosuppressive drugs are cyclosporine and interferon. They are used in refractory lesions in adults who do not respond to any other forms of treatment. The hyperactive immune system of the Atopic Dermatitis patient is controlled by immunosuppressive drugs. They suppress the immune system by inhibiting the production of some antibodies, immune cells and other factors involved in giving exaggerated reactions to the smallest stimuli. They will reduce their action and hence a lower effect of the overactive immune system is seen. The immunosuppressive drugs are employed for a short period of time. They cannot be given for long because a normal immune response is required for the body to resist against various kinds of infection. If they are given for a long time, it may happen that the patient may develop various kinds of respiratory infection, gastric infection, urinary infections, etc. These infections will produce fever, malaise, weakness and other side effects. Immunosuppressive drugs should be used under the strict supervision of an expert dermatologist only. Self-medication of these drugs should never be done as it may cause serious, toxic side effects if used haphazardly.

The common side effects of immunosuppressive drugs include: 1) hypertension (increased blood pressure), 2) gastric complaints like nausea, vomiting; renal (kidney) insufficiencies; central nervous system symptoms like severe headache, tingling and numbness in back and extremities (hands and legs), 3) cancerous growth on skin, 4) acute and chronic infections in various systems of the body, etc. Patients treated with immunosuppressive drugs will be relieved from their symptoms quickly, but the risk of relapse always prevails. The patient may be relieved for only a few weeks to months. It can be concluded that immunosuppressive drugs are not a permanent solution in relieving symptoms. While the patient is taking immunosuppressive drugs, he or she must always remain aware of triggering factors and must remain away from them, as they do not allow the treatment to work efficiently.

The treating physician should also be in search of alternative therapies that may benefit the patient without causing side effects. Efforts are made by the dermatologist to put the patient on a minimal dose of alternative therapy.

5. Need of Hospitalization

In some cases the patient does not respond even to immunosuppressive drugs. These types of cases are extremely rare. These patients have an advanced disease and have been suffering from Atopic Dermatitis for decades. They may have tried all types of treatment but are still not improving. These patients can be benefitted by hospitalization. Hospitalization is required in severe refractory cases not responding to any treatment, and in those cases where secondary infection with microorganisms has penetrated deep inside the body and has caused systemic infection. Symptoms like high-grade fever, nausea, vomiting, diarrhea, dehydration, headache, malaise, severe pain, etc., develop as a result of secondary systemic infections. These toxic symptoms require hospitalization for at least a week. Oral antibiotics, glucose pints, and intravenous pain relievers are given during the hospital stay.

A hospital stay is also required during severely flared-up conditions of Atopic Dermatitis when the whole body is covered with lesions. The patient is generally in great discomfort. In this situation, intensive care in the hospital soothes the lesions greatly. Intensive care in a hospital is also required when the patient is not able to stay away from triggering factors and maintaining causes at home. The patient may be residing or working in such surroundings where he/she is continuously exposed to irritants, allergens, pollutants and other substances that aggravate Atopic Dermatitis. The hospital environment is usually free from all these toxic substances and hence symptoms of the disease are quickly relieved.

There are many patients who are not able to follow the routine skin care regimen advised by the physician. They may be lazy to follow them or they may be in situations/circumstances where they are not able to follow the routine skin care regimen. For example, the physician has advised the patient not to wet his/her hands frequently but the patient washes dishes and cannot follow the regimen due to his/her work. Another example is that a physician has advised an athlete who is involved in outdoor games and is suffering from Atopic Dermatitis to stay out of the harsh sun. Due to the profession, it is not possible to avoid sun and sweat. In such circumstances, if these kinds of patients are admitted to hospital, they will remain away from offending stimuli and will be greatly relieved. The hospital environment also allows the patient to stay away from the day-to-day stress of life. Worries of managing home, office, children, etc., are not present at the hospital and the patient is able to relax. Patients sometimes have a tendency to skip or forget medicines or they may either take an underdose or overdose of the prescribed medicines. The sufficient dose of the medicine may not be received due to haphazard intake of medicines. This can be managed at the hospital, where timely doses are given and no dose is skipped. External applications are applied generously and in the correct amount.

If secondary infections are present, then laboratory investigations are required to be done. It becomes more convenient to conduct investigations, as pathological laboratories are usually present in the hospital. In case of secondary infections, good dressings can be put on the lesions. Regular changing of the dressings are done, which is of great importance in healing the wounds. This is effectively managed in hospitals. Moreover, in the case of secondary infection with Staphylococcus, Streptococcus, S. Aureus, Herpes simplex, Herpes zoster, other fungal infections (Ring worm, etc.), and isolation of the patient is more beneficial. These microorganisms may spread to people in close contact with the patient. A hospital stay quickly clears up infection so that it does not spread to deeper tissues and other healthy persons. Cleanliness is maintained in the hospital and timely bathing and sponging of the patient is done. Under good conditions and surroundings, the symptoms clear up quickly and the result is sustained for a longer period of time. Hence hospitalization in certain situations is very helpful.

6. Causes of Failure of Initial Treatment Regimen and Recurrences

Initial treatment with good skin care and emollients fails in Atopic Dermatitis patients for several reasons. There may be a single reason for recurrence or combination for a variety of reasons. As discussed earlier, Atopic Dermatitis is a periodic disease. There may be periods of flare and periods of remission. If the patient does not improve after conservative therapy, it can be considered that the period of flare is much more severe and stronger in comparison to the treatment employed earlier. The treatment given is weak in comparison to the severity of the disease. Hence the treatment must be revised again. Usually with proper treatment, the majority of patients improve within three weeks, but a few patients do not respond to the treatment as the treatment plan does not suit them and the complete effect is not brought on.

It should be kept in mind that every patient needs to be treated individually. Signs and symptoms in patients vary greatly from one another and hence a common treatment plan cannot be employed for every patient. It may not give a satisfactory result in all the patients of Atopic Dermatitis. Treatment may even fail when the maintaining cause is not addressed in the initial treatment regimen.

Triggering factors may also be overlooked in the initial treatment plan. The commonly found maintaining factors and triggering factors include: 1) emotional imbalance, 2) hormonal imbalance, 3) stress, 4) secondary infection with pathogens, 5) use of medicines that react adversely, 6) continuous exposure to dirt, dust, pollens, pet hairs, dander, etc., 7) use of irritant soaps, perfumes, etc., 8) occupational exposure to chemicals irritants, 9) continuous wetting of hands, 10) living in wet, damp surroundings, 11) exposure to harsh sun, etc. Hence for satisfactory results and visible improvement of the skin, maintaining and triggering factors need to be given equal importance in planning the treatment regimen. Initial treatment may even fail when the patient does not follow the treatment program suggested by the physician. The local ointments given for application may not be regularly applied by the patient. They may even mix the emollient with other local applications and hence the emollient may fail to provide good results. The patient may use harsh, fragrant soaps and deodorants during the course of initial treatment, which deteriorates the skin condition so that the initial treatment with skin care regimen and emollients fails.

7. Is Surgery Required in Atopic Dermatitis?

No, surgery is not required in the Atopic Dermatitis patient. It is a superficial skin disease. It can be well managed with external ointments and internal medicines. Cosmetic surgery is not indicated as the disease can occur and reoccur at any site of the body.

8. Is a cure possible in Atopic Dermatitis?

Yes, a cure is possible in Atopic Dermatitis patients. With age, Atopic Dermatitis usually resolves. In adulthood it is less likely to occur. It can be very well managed with a good skin care regimen and certain precautions. However, the disease may flare up anytime as it is closely related to allergens and irritants present in the environment. Moreover, it has a genetic predisposition and hence reoccurrence can occur.

Chapter 8: How Is Atopic Dermatitis Treated In Infants And Children?

The conservative treatment of infants and children is similar to adults. They are managed with daily skin care routines and aggressive treatment is not required unless signs and symptoms worsen or secondary infection sets in. Atopic lesions usually occur on the face, eyes and surrounding zone in infants and children. Infants and children possess very sensitive and soft skin. In daily skin care routines, the mother is advised to bathe the babies daily with lukewarm water. Very hot or cold water should not be used. Bathing should not be avoided in any circumstances. Sponging with lukewarm water can be done when bathing is not possible. Mothers should not vigorously rub the skin while giving a bath to infants and children. Soap free shower gels or mild baby bars formulated specially for infant skin must be used. After bathing, thick, non-fragrant, chemical free, natural emollient or cream is immediately applied all over the body when the body of the infant is slightly wet. This provides a natural barrier to the baby's skin and prevents drying and itching.

The nails of the infants and children must be trimmed short regularly. If the baby scratches the skin with its fingernails, the lesion may open up and bleeding may occur. Opened lesions are susceptible to secondary infection. The mother can make the children wear gloves, socks or mittens while playing, sleeping, etc., so that they do not scratch directly with the nails. The nails of the mother, family members and babysitters who are handling the baby should be trimmed short and filed smooth. Long nails should not be kept, as they may injure the skin of the baby while bathing, playing or handling the baby.

Clothes should be cautiously selected for children with Atopic Dermatitis. Soft cotton clothes must be preferred. Nylon,

94

polyester and rough material should be avoided. The clothes must be loose fitting and should not stick to the skin. Tight fitting clothes irritate the skin and cause perspiration. Infants and children have the tendency to wet their clothes. Wet clothes should be immediately changed as fungal infection may occur due to constantly wet skin. Bed sheets, napkins, towels etc., used by the infants should be regularly washed and dried. Bed sheets and napkins should be changed if they are wet. Infants and children frequently pass urine and stool. The areas should be immediately cleaned and dried. Soft cotton diapers should be used but they should be frequently changed at regular intervals. Pieces of soft cotton clothes can be used instead of diapers if diaper rashes develop.

The house must be kept thoroughly clean. Regular cleaning should be done so that dirt, dust, dust mites, allergens, pollens, etc., do not accumulate in the house. These offending substances irritate the skin and aggravate itching. It is advisable not to keep pets like dogs or cats in the house as their fur and hair may produce an allergic reaction in children. Pets may lick the skin of infants and children and aggravate Atopic Dermatitis.

The house must be kept cool. The child must not be taken into very hot or cold weather. Direct exposure to harsh sun must be avoided, and if unavoidable, the child must be well protected with soft clothes and a hat. Pleasant surroundings do not cause perspiration and help in relieving itching.

Usually signs and symptoms of Atopic Dermatitis are aggravated at night. The child subconsciously scratches severely at night, hence the lesions become raw. Antihistamines (those substances that suppress the release of histamines in the body that cause itching, redness and swelling) can be given at nighttime before sleep, so that itching is relieved. It is very important for the mother and relatives to recognize the secondary skin infections on the skin of the babies.

If blisters, pustules, oozing pus, crusty or severely inflamed skin are found, a pediatrician or a dermatologist must immediately be consulted and treatment should be started. A child with Atopic Dermatitis is usually irritable, agitated, lonely and restless due to the annoying symptoms of Atopic Dermatitis. The child cries on little matters and may go on to become more demanding. The mother and family members should understand the behavior of the child and should have patience while dealing with the child. Parents and guardians should encourage the child to play and remain with friends and attend school regularly.

Shyness and an inferiority complex usually develop in a child due to the appearance of the skin. Parents should motivate the child that he/she will be quickly relieved from the symptoms. Efforts must be made to distract the attention of the child away from scratching. Whenever scratching is attempted, parents should distract the attention of the child in playing games or towards activities in which the child is interested. In places where a rash appears, a piece of soft cotton cloth or a bandage can be used to cover it. This will not allow the external stimulus to affect the skin. Even the child will not scratch it anymore, as the rashes are not visible to him/her. These factors will improve the skin condition and the child will have a feeling of wellbeing.

In the Case of Infants and Children, the mother can ask the following questions:

- What is the cure rate of the disease?

- How severe is the disease?

- What are the short term and long-term side effects of the treatment?

- What is the effect of treatment on the growth of the child?

- Can the child be allowed to go outdoors and play?

- Can the child be sent to school?

- Can the child be allowed to play with pets?

- Is there any food that is required to be restricted?

- Will the child be relieved temporarily or will there be a flare-up within a few months or years?

- Will the disease continue until adulthood?

- Will there be any effect that can continue until adulthood?

- Is there any way to prevent a flare-up of the disease?

- What vaccination schedule is to be given during treatment?

- Is there any vaccine available for Atopic Dermatitis?

Patients should freely ask these questions to their treating physician. If they do not understand the answers given by the physician, they should ask again for clarification. No confusion should remain about anything related to Atopic Dermatitis. If they do not understand about the skin care regimen and how to take medicines, they should ask it again and should not make any mistake in following the treatment.

The patient may talk to attending nurses about how to take good care at home. If any alternative therapist is present along with the physician, then the patient may ask about available alternative therapy and its benefits for relieving the symptoms.

A patient should never be shy about discussing any problem related to Atopic Dermatitis with the treating physician. No embarrassment should be felt in talking about any personal health issue. If the lesions of Atopic Dermatitis are present on the private parts, the patient should not hesitate to talk about it.

Patients should not even feel shy about undressing (if the skin lesions are present on the private parts) during the physical examination. Patients should openly talk about any disease related to the skin. Any disease present in family members also must be disclosed without hesitation.

No information should be hidden or forgotten. This can harm the patient, as a complete medical history is very much necessary for planning the treatment. If the patient has any bad habits, they must be openly confessed in front of the physician. Bad habits like excessive alcohol consumption, cigarette smoking, drugs, night watching, etc., have great hazards on the health and they may aggravate the signs and symptoms of Atopic Dermatitis. They may even serve as maintaining causes. For example, if the patient has a bad habit of cigarette smoking and he/she suffers from Atopic Dermatitis on the face, then complaints would relapse recurrently, as cigarette smoke irritates the lesions.

A patient should also openly discuss any sensitive issues with the physician. If the patient suffers from any emotional imbalance, he or she should disclose them at the beginning of the treatment. Emotional stress does not have a direct role in Atopic Dermatitis, but it may cause a flare-up of the disease. Patients usually hide complaints as they may be ashamed of them and do not want anyone to know about them. In this case, the family members should convey to the physician about any mental or emotional disturbance of the patient.

Patients should not self-medicate at any time. They should not increase or decrease the prescribed doses of medicines and external applications. They should not omit or add any medicines or topical applications. Before making any changes in the prescribed treatment, the patient should contact the treating physician. The patient should either personally visit or call up the physician before making any changes. If any medicine or external application does not suit, then the patient should immediately contact the physician but should not discontinue the medicine unless ordered to by the physician. Patients should also not discontinue treatments if they are completely relieved of the signs and symptoms.

Patients might be tempted to stop the medicines in between the course of treatment when lesions have disappeared completely, but this should not be done because if the treatment is not adequately completed, then the disease may flare up at any time. Relief will be obtained only temporarily and chances of a relapse are increased. Patients may even discontinue the medicines when they have taken medicines for a long period of time and found no improvement. The patient may get frustrated and discontinues the medicines, but this should not be done since certain severe lesions of Atopic Dermatitis may take a long time to heal. Some medicines also take a long time to show their effect. The patient should keep patience. They must follow the physician and should not interfere in treatment. Patients should also always consult the treating doctor before starting any alternative therapy.

If the treating physician allows adding an alternative therapy, only then should the patient start them, as certain drugs used in alternative therapy may interact with other ongoing treatment. They may either reduce or exaggerate the effect of the ongoing therapy. Lesions may get worse or they may develop some new signs or symptoms due to the effect of alternative therapy. This can confuse the treating physician about the presenting signs and symptoms. It may happen that the physician may add some more medicines or may omit medicines, as the presenting picture of the disease has changed. Alternative therapies like Ayurveda, Homoeopathy, Unani, Chinese herbs, etc., should always be used only after consulting with the treating physician. Patients should also never mix any cosmetic products with the prescribed external applications. The medicinal properties of the prescribed external application may be reduced when combined with harsh, chemical based cosmetics.

Chapter 9: Treating Contact Dermatitis Naturally

1. Home remedies

Various kinds of home remedies are used for treating Atopic Dermatitis. They can be used along with the main line of treatment. They are easy to use. The ingredients used in home remedies are easily available in grocery stores and in your own kitchen. They help in soothing the skin and reducing itching and scratching. They protect the skin against the irritants present in the surrounding environment. The majority of home remedies provide symptomatic relief of itching, swelling, rashes, etc. Home remedies must be used only after consulting the treating physician as they may interact with the prescribed medicines and external applications.

They may not allow the prescribed medicines to work and may alter their effect. Although home remedies are very mild and usually do not cause any side effects, they should be used only under the supervision of the treating physician and allergist. All the pros and cons of the home remedies must be well researched before commencing its use.

The commonly used home remedies are as follows:

1) Coconut oil - Pure coconut oil can be applied regularly on the sites of the lesions as well as over the whole body. The skin quickly absorbs coconut oil. It can be used twice a day. It can be gently massaged all over the body before bathing. It should be left on the skin for 20 minutes, then a bath can be taken with gentle, soap-free cleanser. Coconut oil helps to keep the skin soft and nourished. The natural oil of the skin is preserved and dryness is prevented.

2) Spearmint leaves - Spearmint leaves are crushed with water

and a fine paste is made. This paste is applied over the skin where severe itching, rashes or inflammation is found. It can be applied once a day. The paste helps in relieving inflammation and quick healing of the lesions is seen.

3) Papaya seeds- Papaya seeds are meshed with water or natural oil and a fine paste is made. It is rubbed gently over the affected skin. It can be used twice a week. It serves as a gentle scrub and helps in relieving the severe itch. It heals the lesion faster.

4) Licorice root, calendula flower and ginkgo can be crushed and applied on the skin. They are effective in controlling inflammation.

5) Chamomile, witch hazel extract, borage seed oil, chickweed, squalene and vegetable glycerine can be applied on the lesions of Atopic Dermatitis. They soothe the skin and prevent dryness.

Along with home remedies, the patient can take care of the skin at home by following certain simple methods, which will prevent skin irritation.

Always wash new clothes before wearing them for the first time. New clothes are treated with formaldehyde, dyes and other chemical irritants, which can irritate the skin and aggravate itching. Washing removes these irritants. Always wash the clothes with abundant water. Rinse the clothes thoroughly so that soap and detergents do not remain on them. It is preferable to rinse the clothes twice. Always use a mild laundry detergent that is a non- irritant for the hands and skin.

Always wear loose, smooth textured, cotton clothes. If one does not like cotton clothes then cotton blend clothes or clothes prepared from other natural fabrics can be used. Clothes that remain away from the skin and do not constantly touch the skin should be worn. Very tight clothes do not allow the skin to breathe and increase perspiration, which irritates the lesions. Woolen and leather clothes should be totally avoided. Airy clothes must be used during exercise so that excessive perspiration does not occur and is absorbed faster by the clothes if it does occur.

Avoid using woolen and nylon bedding so that excessive perspiration does not occur at night and friction is not created with the skin. It will prevent night itching of the skin.

Fingernails should always be trimmed short and filed smooth so that scratching hard with long nails is prevented.

Always have a bath with lukewarm water for 10-15 minutes. Long baths should not be taken. Mild, soap-free, gentle cleansers can be used for bathing. Enough water should be used in bathing. No residual soap or cleanser should remain on the skin, especially in the folds of the skin. Baking soda, crushed oatmeal (uncooked), or colloidal oatmeal (oatmeal crushed to fine powder and used especially for bathing only), bath salts, etc., can be added to lukewarm water. They serve as a mild scrub, which removes dead skin and flakes from the lesions. Harsh scrubs should be totally avoided.

Two to three tablespoons of bleach can also be added to bathing water. It is preferable to use it diluted. Diluted bleach does not allow various pathogens to grow on the skin, and thus secondary infection can be prevented. Bathing in a swimming pool is to be avoided. If it is unavoidable, one can have a short bath in a swimming pool, followed immediately by a fresh water bath. After bathing, emollients are to be applied on the skin, which will seal in the moisture of the skin. Moisturizers and emollients can be applied twice a day after bathing, in the morning and before going to bed. Moisturizers containing vitamin B12 are preferable. They should be generously applied over the legs, arms, back and the folds of the skin.

Always apply sunscreen before leaving the house. Sunscreen can be chosen according to the harshness of the sun in the surrounding area and the sensitivity of the skin. Sunscreen of SPF 15 or higher is advisable. It provides protection against UVA and UVB rays, which irritates the skin.

Try to keep a constant temperature and humidity indoors. Abrupt alterations in the surrounding temperature and humidity can irritate the skin. The air inside the house is usually dry and hot. It lacks the necessary humidity and moisture suitable for sensitive skin. Hot, dry and low humidity air causes irritation to the skin and leads to itching, burning, scaling and parching of the skin. In these conditions, a home humidifier can be used. Portable home humidifiers are readily available. They can be placed in the room. Various types of humidifiers are available according to the requirements of the person. Humidifiers must be hygienically maintained; otherwise they can harbor a variety of microorganisms like bacteria and fungi. The growth of microorganisms increases in high humidity conditions.

Avoid taking stale and tinned food. These foods contain high amounts of preservatives, irritants and allergens, which irritate the skin. Instead, take fresh, natural and homemade food. Soya products, eggs, sour fruits, meat, etc., can cause allergic reactions and hence should be avoided. A diet rich in essential fatty acids can be very helpful in healing the lesions. Walnuts, almonds, cashew nuts, primrose oil, fish oil, sunflower seeds and other seeds are rich in essential fatty acids. They can be consumed in the required amounts daily. Supplements of vitamin A, vitamin E and zinc should be consumed along with essential fatty acids. These supplements prevent nutritional deficiencies and make the skin healthier. Healthy skin can withstand allergens and irritants more effectively. Primrose oil, when consumed daily, shows great improvement in skin symptoms in children without causing any side effects. Primrose oil is given daily for 4-20 weeks.

In the case of severe itching, a cool, wet bandage or cloth can be tied on the affected site. It will soothe the skin and prevent scratching. Calamine lotion or an anti-itch cream can be applied on the skin for soothing effect. Over the counter products like one percent hydrocortisone cream can also be helpful. Oral antihistamines like diphenhydramine (Benadryl) can be taken at nighttime when the itching is severe. It relieves itching and causes drowsiness.

Avoid unnecessary stress at home and at work. To combat against stress, meditation, yoga, breathing exercises and relaxation therapy can be practiced daily. Massage therapy can be useful in relieving stress. It increases circulation on the skin surface and helps in faster healing. Behavior modification techniques can be learned from a psychologist. They help in controlling anger and frustration arising from severe itching.

2. Chinese medicine

Chinese therapy can be used by many Atopic Dermatitis patients. Chinese therapy includes Chinese medicines, acupuncture treatment, dietary alterations and Chinese topical creams. Chinese herbal tea is commonly used as a Chinese medicine. It is made by boiling the Chinese herbs for a certain time (usually for one hour). Dried herbs are used in it. They are allowed to remain in hot water for some time and then drained. This medicinal water is consumed in the morning on an empty stomach. These herbs have healing properties, which heal the lesions faster. Acupuncture treatment activates the healing system of the skin and reduces inflammation. Chinese therapy is not useful for all patients. Every individual patient requires different therapy. Chinese therapy can cause liver, kidney and heart toxicities. Hence, it should be taken only after consulting an expert Chinese therapist and the treating physician.

3. Herbal medicine

Herbal medicines that purify the liver, nervous system and blood can be used for healing the lesions. The herbal medicines have a detoxifying effect on the body. Toxins like heavy elements, drug materials, allergens, irritants, etc., accumulate in the body and are removed in detoxification. They help to purify the body from within and reduce the hypersensitivity of the skin. The common detoxifying tonics and purifiers include burdock, red clover, etc. Burdock is a liver tonic and a purifier. It helps the normal functioning of the liver and removes toxins from the liver. It is very helpful for patients having Atopic Dermatitis along with addiction of alcohol and poor liver function. It also benefits Atopic Dermatitis patients with fatty liver (accumulation of fat in the liver). The thick syrup of Burdock is mixed with water and is consumed daily in the morning on an empty stomach.

Red clover helps purify the blood and remove allergens and irritants that cause itching and rashes. It is also available in syrup form, which is diluted with water and consumed in the morning on an empty stomach.

Topical herbal creams are freely available on the market. They are not 100% herbal and contain corticosteroids in them. Long-term use of corticosteroids can cause side effects like excessive hair on the body, thin skin, rough skin, stretch marks, etc. Herbal creams show instant result due to the steroid in them. They should be carefully used as they may cause contact dermatitis in the patient.

4. Ayurvedic medicine

The Ayurvedic system of medicine is an ancient system of medicine from India. It has been widely used all over the world for centuries. It is a 100% natural system of medicine and uses leaves, roots, flowers, bark, etc., for the preparation of medicines. It is a non-invasive method, and has no side effects.

The medicines are given in oral form as tablets, crushed powders and syrups. The local applications are given in paste form or as ointments.

Some of the Ayurvedic medicines used for Atopic Dermatitis are as follows:

Margosa leaves (neem leaves) are crushed to a fine paste (approximate 1 tbs) and turmeric powder (approximate 1tsp) is added to it. It is mixed well and is applied twice a day on the lesions. Margosa leaves and turmeric powder are considered as natural antiseptics and help in faster healing of the lesions. Turmeric powder and margosa leaves (leaves are dried and fine powder is made) can also be taken orally. It is advisable to consume it daily early in the morning on an empty stomach. It purifies the body from within.

50 grams of margosa leaves are added to 200 grams of mustard oil and the mixture is heated. The oil is heated until the margosa leaves turn black. Then the oil is cooled down overnight and is strained the next day. This neem oil can be applied 3 times a day on the affected site. It is advisable to apply it for 1 year. It soothes the skin, prevents dryness and provides an antiseptic effect. It prevents recurrence and flare-up of the lesions.

Fresh aloe vera leaves are peeled off and the gel within the leaves is removed. The gel is applied directly on the lesions and is left on for 30 minutes. It can be applied daily. It has soothing properties and it relieves severe itching, burning and dryness of the skin. It is advisable to use only fresh aloe vera gel and not the packed ones available on the market made with preservatives.

5. Homeopathic medicine

Homeopathic treatment is an effective alternative treatment with no side effects that are commonly found with conventional therapy. Homeopathy has proven very effective in both short term and long-term management of Atopic Dermatitis. Homeopathic philosophy believes in treating the person as a whole instead of treating localized signs and symptoms. It corrects the body from within and removes the disease completely. A homeopathic system of medicine does not palliate the signs and symptoms. It cures them. This modern system treats the individual and not the disease.

Various homeopathic medicines are used for the treatment of Atopic Dermatitis. They are given on the basis of individual signs and symptoms of the patient and not the common symptoms of the disease. For example, common signs and symptoms of Atopic Dermatitis are severe itching, scratching, burning, rashes, etc., but the individual signs and symptoms are itching aggravated only during the day and relieved at nighttime, scratching until bleeding, burning only in the head area, feet and hands, rashes relieved by cold baths, etc. A homeopathic physician gives medicine on the basis of the individual symptoms.

Constitutional medicines are given on the basis of man as a whole. The individual signs and symptoms of the disease, aggravating factors, ameliorating factors, likes, dislikes, food habits, thirst, bowel habits, mental and emotional state, etc., are all considered before prescribing the constitutional medicine. The causative factor, personal history, family history, etc., of the patient is thoroughly investigated and only then is medicine prescribed. In the case of a female, menstrual history, pregnancy, birth history of the baby, etc., are inquired about. Some of the examples of constitutional medicines that are given after considering all the above factors are sulphur, Natrum mur, Thuja, Siphilinum, etc.

In the case of infants and children, parents and guardians are interviewed for the above information, as the children cannot narrate the individual signs and symptoms. Parents can narrate the causative factors, aggravating factors, ameliorating factors, onset of symptoms, etc., of the child. With the help of thorough case taking, the link between the various events of the child's life and the disease is established by the homeopathic physician. The various events of life, such as separation from parents, births of siblings, strained relations with parents, new residing place, introduction of new foods, accidents, etc., are all inquired about as they can become the triggering factors for Atopic Dermatitis. Medicines are prescribed on the basis of these events. For example, Natrum mur medicine works very well when a child develops Atopic Dermatitis after a separation from the mother. Another example is Pulsatilla, which works well when the signs and symptoms begin during puberty.

Constitutional medicines provide long-term relief and correct the body from within. In circumstances where constitutional medicines cannot be given or when the patient requires immediate relief in an acute phase, therapeutic medicines are also given.

Localized signs and symptoms are taken into consideration when prescribing therapeutic medicines. These medicines provide quick, short-term relief. The common examples of therapeutic medicines are as follows:

Graphitis: It is given when the eczema is crusty and oozing. Sticky fluid oozes out and the skin is cracked.

Sulphur: It is given when severe burning, redness, and inflammation is found on the skin, which is aggravated by bathing and hot weather. The eruptions are red, scaly, crusted, dry or moist. It works very well when all other medications and ointments have failed to give satisfactory results.

Antimonium crudum: It is given when the skin is thick and cracked. Indigestion and obesity usually accompany the skin problems. The eczema symptoms like itching become worse after eating pickles, vinegar and sour food, and after heat and sun exposure. Adult patients are usually sensitive and sentimental and the children are shy and irritable.

Arsenicum album: It is given when the eczema is dry and burning. Severe itching and scratching is found, which is relieved by applying heat and hot fomentation. The person becomes very anxious and restless due to the disease and itching. Indigestion and chilliness accompanies eczema. The patient is very neat, orderly and clean.

Arum triphyllum: It is given when the eczema and the allergic skin eruptions are found on the lower part of the face, mouth, chin, lips, nostrils etc. The skin is chapped, hot, irritated, cracked and raw. The patient has the habit of picking the lips due to which they become raw. Throat irritation and hoarseness accompanies skin symptoms.

Calcarea carbonica: It is given when the eczematous skin is cracked. The skin symptoms are worse in the winter season and cold surroundings. The patient is exhausted, anxious and overwhelmed due to skin symptoms. Obesity and sluggish metabolism accompanies the skin symptoms. The patient is very chilly and has cold, clammy hands and feet.

Calendula: Calendula is applied when the skin is irritated, inflamed and infected. Calendula is available in ointment, lotion, gel, or tincture form. It has soothing and healing properties.

Graphites: It is given when the skin disorders like impetigo, herpes, and eczema have been present for a long time. The skin of the patient is tough, leathery, cracked and sore. The lesions are found on and around the ears, mouth, or hands. The eczema is cracked and crusty with a golden discharge. Itching of the skin is aggravated from the warmth of the bed and the patient scratches the skin until it bleeds.

Hepar sulphuris calcareum: It is given when the eczema is sore and infected. The skin is chapped, cracked, and the lesions take a very long time to heal. The patients are sensitive, chilly, vulnerable and irritable.

Mezereum: It is given when the eruptions and blisters ooze and form thick crusts. The skin is thick with severe itching that is relived by cold applications and open air. The patient is anxious and has a craving for fat.

Rhus toxicodendron: It is given when the eczema is red, swollen and has blister-like eruptions. Severe itching is found, which is relieved by heat and hot applications. The person becomes restless, irritable and anxious due to the itching and eczema. Muscle stiffness may accompany skin symptoms.

Petroleum: It is given when the skin is very dry, cracked, sore, infected, tough and leathery due to long-term irritation. Eczematous skin is deeply sore and cracked, which is aggravated in winter and cold surroundings. Itching and scratching is worse at night due to the warmth of the bed. A cold sensation is felt after itching and scratching. The lesions are found on the fingertips and palms.

The Dosage and the Repetition of Therapeutic medicines:

Initially, the therapeutic treatment is started with lower potencies like 6X, 6C, 12X, 12C, 30X, or 30C

After giving one dose, the physician usually waits for a response and if improvement is found, the dose is not repeated. Dosing is repeated only when further improvement ceases. The dose is repeated according to the requirement. It may be given hourly, daily, monthly or even annually. The frequency of repetition of the dose is decided on the basis of the condition of the patient and the severity of the disease.

A new medicine is given only when no response is found from the previously prescribed medicine.

6. Probiotic (harmless live bacteria) dietary supplements.

Probiotics are recommended, along with the external applications, for many people. Probiotics are naturally available from curd and buttermilk. They are also available in tablets and granule form. They are believed to reduce lesions, especially in children. The exact mechanism, blend and amount of probiotic required for reducing the lesion are not known. Patients must contact their treating physician before starting it, as it may interact with ongoing therapy or may induce allergic reactions. The patient should ask the physician or alternate therapist to prescribe the right probiotic and in the correct dose if they feel it would work beneficially to heal lesions.

Dietary supplements containing vitamin E, vitamin B6, Borage oil, zinc, etc., are used for relieving lesions, but have not been thoroughly proven.

Green tea, black tea and oolong tea are believed to reduce the allergic reactions in the body. They may improve the body's immune system. They can be consumed many times a day. In some patients they have shown significant results in reducing lesions, but in some patients no beneficial effect is noticed. These teas contain caffeine, which can increase sleeplessness, anxiety and restlessness in the patient. Hence it should be used only after consulting the treating physician.

Chamomile tea can cause severe allergic reactions and anaphylaxis, (severe allergic reaction of the body in which the blood pressure falls, breathing becomes difficult, unconsciousness is found and a person may die). Hence it is preferable to avoid chamomile tea.

Alternative treatment should be taken under the strict supervision of an expert alternative therapist and only after consulting the treating physician. It should be kept in mind that alternative treatments are only supportive treatments. They cannot substitute for the conventional treatment given for healing the lesions. Patients can take alternative treatments along with the main line of treatment after consulting the physician. Any change or reaction encountered after the use of alternative medicines and ointments should be conveyed to the physician right away.

Chapter 10: How To Control And Prevent Atopic Dermatitis

For controlling Atopic Dermatitis, the patient should follow the daily skin care regimen prescribed by the physician. Harsh soaps, harsh cleansers, makeup removers, astringents, etc., should not be used. These agents drain away the natural moisture and oil that is required for healthy skin. After bathing, moisturizing creams and emollients must be applied. They should be applied twice a day. Waterproof emollients are preferred. Patients should make a habit of applying emollients after hand washing and face washing. This will prevent drying and stretching of the skin. Lotions are generally not recommended due to their liquid consistency. Thick emollients make a coating over the skin, which will prevent direct exposure to allergens and irritants. The skin will remain protected due to this barrier.

Whenever the patient feels the urge to scratch, it should be resisted. The patient should avoid scratching and rubbing harshly. Instead of scratching with fingernails, a soft cotton cloth can be used for rubbing the skin. A soft cotton cloth will relieve the itch and will prevent the "itch- scratch" cycle. Bleeding will also be prevented, which usually occurs when the patient scratches with long nails. Fingernails of adults and children should be trimmed short and filed smooth.

Patients should not wet their hands very often. Frequent face washing is also not recommended. Washing the face only two or three times a day is recommended. The skin should be protected against the irritants by avoiding them. Contact with the following general irritants should be avoided: 1) harsh sun, 2) polluted surroundings containing harmful gases like carbon dioxide, carbon monoxide, hydrogen sulphide, etc., 3) harsh water containing excess chlorine, 4) sea water, 5) use of low quality, harsh makeup and cosmetics, 6) harsh deodorants, 7) perfumed soaps, 8) rough clothes like polyester or nylon, 9) tight clothes, 10) wearing artificial jewellery (which may cause constant irritation and friction), etc., should be avoided. Exposure to dust, animal dander, fur and hair, dirt, dust mites, etc., should be avoided as far as possible. If it is not possible to avoid them completely, then one should limit exposure. Use of gloves, handkerchiefs, long sleeved shirts, goggles, scarves, etc., can be helpful in limiting exposure to these irritants. Patients should remain well protected while going outdoors, during travelling and while cleaning the house or office. The use of high quality sun block should be undertaken while travelling in the sun. Patients should ask their physicians to prescribe a good sunscreen that can provide protection against UVA and UVB rays. The use of sunscreen must be preferred over sunscreen lotion. It is advisable to apply the cream 20 minutes before going into the sun.

Patients should contact their physicians when any external application does not suit them or shows allergic reactions.

Patients should always prefer staying indoors and in cool surroundings. Excessive heat will irritate the skin and cause redness and perspiration. Itching will increase in hot weather. Patients should prefer staying in steady humidity levels. Leaving on air conditioners at home and in the office and then suddenly going into the hot sun outside should be avoided. Patients should not have an immediate bath after coming in from outdoors where there is extreme heat and after excessive perspiration. This can cause sudden changes in the core temperature of the body, which is not suitable for the patient.

Patients must avoid unnecessary stress at work and in routine matters. Excess stress leads to constant anxiety, which may flare up the lesions. Patients must learn to keep calm and feel relaxed. They must also learn to identify the factors that cause stress and anxiety and must keep away from them. Peace of mind helps the patient to recover faster. Meditation and relaxation techniques can be very helpful to prevent anxiety and depression related to itching and appearance.

In the case of babies, to control Atopic Dermatitis, breastfeeding should be promoted. Breast milk does not cause any allergies and contains protective antibodies that fight against microorganisms. Breastfeeding should be given until one-and-a-half years of age. Until six months of age, only breast milk must be given. There is no requirement for any other food. After six months, solid food can be started gradually after consulting the treating physician. Any food that can cause allergies like eggs, soya milk, etc., must be avoided. Thus, by practicing the above-discussed points, Atopic Dermatitis can be easily controlled in adults and children.

Is There any Vaccine Available for Atopic Dermatitis?

No vaccine is available for Atopic Dermatitis. Other vaccines should be taken after consulting the pediatrician and dermatologist. The small pox vaccine should not be taken by a patient with mild or severe Atopic Dermatitis. It can flare up the lesions. It should not even be taken by people who are currently healthy with no lesions, but have been diagnosed with Atopic Dermatitis previously. The disease can reactivate and serious complications can occur. Patients with Atopic Dermatitis also should not come in close contact with persons who have been recently vaccinated with the small pox vaccine. Close contact with bed sheets, clothes, soaps and other items used by the vaccinated person must be avoided, as these items can also aggravate and infect the lesions.

Physical contact with the site of vaccination should also be avoided until the scab falls off (the wound heals and the scab falls off after approximately three weeks). If contact is unavoidable, then the site of the vaccine must be covered with a cloth or bandage. If new rashes develop and unusual signs or symptoms occur, the patient should immediately contact the treating physician. Small pox has now been eradicated in the majority of the world's countries, but still, if any patient of Atopic Dermatitis is exposed to a small pox epidemic, then the vaccine can be given under the strict supervision of the physician and dermatologist.

Chapter 11: Self Help Information

Having Atopic Dermatitis is really a terrible experience if the initial treatment fails to resolve the symptoms. Atopic Dermatitis is a problem that is faced not only by children but also by adults, as the previous chapters of this book have explained. Many a times it is an easily preventable problem, but because of it being common or sometimes misdiagnosed, the condition worsens and becomes more complicated than what it really is. It is therefore important to bear in mind that no matter how simple this problem seems to be, timely and effective treatment should always be started to prevent you or your family from suffering further from this condition.

What is the cost of the treatment for Atopic Dermatitis?

The cost of the treatment for Atopic Dermatitis per year is similar to psoriasis, emphysema, epilepsy etc. Managing an Atopic Dermatitis patient is very difficult. Stress is greatly increased on the family since more time is required to be given for caring for the patient, the job of the patient or the family members may be lost, sleep disturbances are commonly encountered by the patient and family members due to night aggravation of the disease and the financial cost of the treatment is also higher.

Great financial losses may be encountered since the disease usually begins in early childhood. The treatment cost of a child suffering from Atopic Dermatitis may be more than a child having type 1 diabetes mellitus. The prevalence rate of Atopic Dermatitis is also increasing day by day in infants as well as in adults. The financial cost greatly increases, as the patient needs to recurrently visit the physician, the allergist and the family physician. The patient may need to be hospitalized, due to which the financial burden increases. The patient needs to regularly visit nurses, pharmacists, dieticians, and psychologists etc, which enhance the treatment cost. The patient may even need to take alternative therapies like homeopathy, ayurveda, and herbal therapy, which contribute to the financial burden. The national *cost of Atopic Dermatitis* is estimated to be $0.9 to 3.8 billion every year in the United States. According to a survey, the individual patient cost of the treatment may be as high as $4,635 in the United States, out of which the medical cost is approx $487, hospital cost approx $2,213, other direct cost approx $954, other indirect cost approx US$980. Nationally, the cost of the treatment of childhood Atopic Dermatitis was around $364 million in the United States in 1990, and $721 million £444 million) in the United Kingdom in 1996.

A patient suffering from Atopic Dermatitis usually becomes irritable, restless and anxious due to the chronic nature of the disease. The patient feels ashamed of the appearance of the skin Itching and scratching of the skin becomes bothersome for the patient. Severe, uncontrolled itching in public places puts the patient into an awkward situation in front of surrounding people. Severe itching also troubles the patient at night and hence sound sleep is prevented. Long continued treatment and restrictions of the disease also irritate the patient. All these negative emotions affect the patient to a great extent and the quality of life may be spoiled due to the disease. Chronic depression and inferiority complex may develop in the patient, which can again worsen the lesions or flare up the acute attacks.

In these circumstances, social forums, educational programmes and awareness sessions become very helpful. They resolve the social issues, queries and confusions of the patient. These programmes are conducted by a physician, non-government organizations, government organizations, private societies etc. Online aid can be obtained from the various societies and firms that are involved in the activities for the betterment of the Atopic Dermatitis patient. These organisations provide answers to numerous queries that the patient may have, which are missed out during the physician's visit or left unanswered. Some of the physicians also run online portals, which provide basic consultation and education to the patient. It is very useful as the patient is able to take help anytime without requiring physical presence. The knowledge and the awareness of the patient about the disease is greatly increased by attending educational programmes and awareness sessions held offline and online.

The patient must attend events organised by physicians and social forums. These events encourage the patient a lot as they meet people with similar sufferings and learn more to combat the disease. Success stories of patients who have completely recovered from Atopic Dermatitis motivate the patient to take timely medicines, follow required precautions and remain calm during the acute phase of the disease. Hearing, knowing and understanding about complaints of other people relieves the patient a lot. The patient can even share their sufferings with people having similar complaints. They can also share tips on how to relieve symptoms. This way, many patients can be benefitted as they may find new, effective ways of relieving signs and symptoms. Mentally, the patient feels confident, relaxed and relieved after communicating with people with similar sufferings and attending help forums and educational and awareness programmes.

Help can be obtained from the following websites:

http://www.worldallergy.org

http://www.patient.co.uk / http://www.allergyuk.org

http://www.britishskinfoundation.org.uk

http://www.britishhomeopathic.org

http://www.britayurpractitioners.com

http://www.topix.com

http://www.medicinenet.com

Conclusion

The skin is the outermost and the most widespread organ of the body, which covers the whole body. The skin protects the body against heat, cold, pollution and surrounding offensive agents. For healthy functioning of the skin and to prevent skin diseases, it must be protected against harmful agents and it must be given adequate nutrition.

The exact cause of Atopic Dermatitis is not known. The disease may be caused due to genetic factors, surrounding environmental factors and a hyperactive immune system of the patient. Weakened immunity predisposes to Atopic Dermatitis. Mutation in the gene involved in the production of filagrin protein, which is found in the epidermis of the skin, predisposes to the development of Atopic Dermatitis.

Atopic Dermatitis may be inherited. It is commonly found in first relatives of the patient, but it may also occur without family history of the disease. It may be associated with other allergic reactions of the body like asthma, hay fever (sneezing, fever, water from the eyes), chronic dermatitis etc. Pathogenesis of asthma, hay fever etc is similar to Atopic Dermatitis. Patients usually have personal and family history of asthma, hay fever and chronic dermatitis.

Infants and young children are commonly affected with Atopic Dermatitis but it can occur in adults and older people too. Infants usually get affected with Atopic Dermatitis around 1 ½ to 3 months of age. At around 4 months of age, the lesions usually resolve but these infants may suffer from dry skin or hand eczema in adulthood. The disease may be localised to any one part of the body or may be generalised. The patient may have periods of flare-ups and remissions. The disease usually clears up with age

119

but few patients may develop the disease in adulthood also. Adults suffer from the disease due to the use of harsh chemicals, soaps, deodorants, cosmetics etc

The symptoms of the Atopic Dermatitis consist of the following:

Inflammation of the skin is found.

Rashes of the disease cover the whole body or some parts of the body.

The skin is itchy, inflamed, red, swollen, dry, cracked, oozing, crusty, and scaly with blister and vesicle formation.

The most common complains are of dry, red and extremely itchy skin and scratching.

Patients of Atopic Dermatitis develop "itch- scratch" cycle where severe itching leads to scratching and scratching again aggravates itching.

Some patients develop lichenification where thick, leathery and dry skin occurs due to constant scratching. Lichenification occurs in the later chronic stage of the disease. Cataract may occur due to Atopic Dermatitis.

Atopic Dermatitis is not a contagious skin disease.

Caution must be taken when a secondary infection with bacteria, virus or fungi has occurred on the lesions.

Diagnostic tools like physical examination, visual inspection and observation of the skin are done by the dermatologist to diagnose Atopic Dermatitis. A thorough personal and family history of the patient is taken. Allergy tests like skin allergy test, blood allergy test, food allergy test etc are done to detect the allergens that trigger off or aggravate the disease.

Conclusion

Certain methods or practices can be adopted that can reduce the exposure to allergens, yet the success of the treatment plan greatly depends on how carefully the patient and family members follow instructions.

A cure is possible for Atopic Dermatitis, and with age it usually resolves. This condition can be very well managed with a good skin care regimen and certain precautions. Atopic Dermatitis does not have effect on quality of life, ignorance can simply cause the patient more discomfort than necessary.

Remember to always consult a doctor before making any changes to your skin care regime or medication. All you have to do is take the right measures to prevent, avoid and cure Atopic Dermatitis and you will find the symptoms ease considerably.

Thank you for reading my book. I hope you've enjoyed it.

Robert Rymore

Published by IMB Publishing 2014

Copyright and Trademarks: This publication is Copyrighted 2014 by IMB Publishing. All products, publications, software and services mentioned and recommended in this publication are protected by trademarks. In such instance, all trademarks & copyright belong to the respective owners. All rights reserved. No part of this book may be reproduced or transferred in any form or by any means, graphic, electronic, or mechanical, including photocopying, recording, taping, or by any information storage retrieval system, without the written permission of the authors. Pictures used in this book are either royalty free pictures bought from stock-photo websites or have the source mentioned underneath the picture.

Disclaimer and Legal Notice: This product is not legal or medical advice and should not be interpreted in that manner. You need to do your own due-diligence to determine if the content of this product is right for you. The author and the affiliates of this product are not liable for any damages or losses associated with the content in this product. While every attempt has been made to verify the information shared in this publication, neither the author nor the affiliates assume any responsibility for errors, omissions or contrary interpretation of the subject matter herein. Any perceived slights to any specific person(s) or organization(s) are purely unintentional. We have no control over the nature, content and availability of the web sites listed in this book. The inclusion of any web site links does not necessarily imply a recommendation or endorse the views expressed within them. IMB Publishing takes no responsibility for, and will not be liable for, the websites being temporarily unavailable or being removed from the Internet. The accuracy and completeness of information provided herein and opinions stated herein are not guaranteed or warranted to produce any particular results, and the advice and strategies, contained herein may not be suitable for every individual. The author shall not be liable for any loss incurred as a consequence of the use and application, directly or indirectly, of any information presented in this work. This publication is designed to provide information in regards to the subject matter covered. The information included in this book has been compiled to give an overview of the subject s and detail some of the symptoms, treatments etc. that are available to people with this condition. It is not intended to give medical advice. For a firm diagnosis of your condition, and for a treatment plan suitable for you, you should consult your doctor or consultant. The writer of this book and the publisher are not responsible for any damages or negative consequences following any of the treatments or methods highlighted in this book. Website links are for informational purposes and should not be seen as a personal endorsement; the same applies to the products detailed in this book. The reader should also be aware that although the web links included were correct at the time of writing, they may become out of date in the future

www.ingramcontent.com/pod-product-compliance
Lightning Source LLC
Chambersburg PA
CBHW060617210326
41520CB00010B/1372

9 7 8 1 9 1 0 4 1 0 6 2 2